HEALTHY AND LEAN

The Science of Metabolism and the
Psychology of Weight Management

Here's to a lifetime of health and happiness! Ileana Riverón

Heidi Wohlrabe, M.D., and Ileana Riverón

ISBN: 978-1-4834-5699-7 (sc)
ISBN: 978-1-4834-5698-0 (e)

Library of Congress Control Number: 2016913253

Lulu Publishing Services rev. date: 10/6/2016

CONTENTS

PREFACE

Heidi Wohlrabe, MD

I am many things: a physician, a mom, a girl, a middle-aged woman, a grandma, a wife, a homemaker, a Christian, an amateur artist, a wannabe ballerina, a frustrated pianist, and a board-certified psychiatrist. Though I have been comfortable balancing various roles in my life, I have never considered myself a writer. However, everyone's life takes unexpected twists and turns, and mine brought me to a point where I could no longer keep silent.

This book was conceived during the period of my life in which I was simultaneously directing an eating disorders clinic and trying to run a home with three young children. While I loved the work I did at my clinic and treasured the time I spent with patients, I found that I was a broken record, reiterating the same educational information week after week. I desperately wanted to get to the point where I was truly listening and doing therapy, not just teaching.

I taught my patients about the flaws of the diets they saw being advertised in magazines, on TV, and even by the United States Department of Agriculture (USDA); the damaging consequences of dieting in general; the medicinal benefits of health foods; the road to a healthy and fast metabolism; and the necessary steps to physical and psychological recovery from disordered eating. I knew that if my patients first understood the science behind their disorder, they would be able to align their own personal goals with the goals of therapy. Then we could both venture toward health together, as a team.

The alignment of goals and the establishment of a trusting doctor-patient bond are essential for effective medical treatment.

Unfortunately, these goals were difficult to achieve in our clinic. Our patients felt successful and psychologically safe when they were in control of their own diets and when they felt thin. The nurses and dietitians, however, felt safe when our patients religiously followed the government-prescribed food pyramid and when they were *pleasingly plump*; after all, plump is always preferable to emaciated or dead.

The fears of the staff were warranted. Eating disorders *are* serious and deadly, and health-care professionals who are monitoring the recovery of eating-disordered patients must take great care to prevent a lapse or relapse into anorexia. Furthermore, the path to recovery from anorexia includes a difficult transition period in which patients need to allow their bodies to do the very thing they fear most: gain a moderate amount of weight in order to compensate for past dieting and starvation behavior. In my view, it was our job to help patients through this especially challenging period by offering them a long-term plan that promised healthy weight stability.

Our recovering patients needed to know that we valued their concerns so they could recover a sense of security. Additionally, they needed to learn what a *safe* lean weight is—one where their body fat never drops below 18 percent for women and 7 percent for men. The food pyramid diet achieved none of these goals. Instead, it merely fed into our patients' fears of long-term weight gain and made treatment a constant patient-staff struggle rather than the partnership it was meant to be.

For rejecting the USDA guidelines, I was seen as a heretic. It took fifteen years for the world to accept the dietary recommendations that I was making back in the nineties. Meanwhile, I grew more and more frustrated by the absence of educational material that would benefit my patients, and I ruminated over the futility of trying to reach people *after* they were already struggling with a serious disease.

Eventually, I closed the clinic in order to give my family my undivided attention but with the intention of returning to work when life slowed down. It never did. (It never does.) Nevertheless, it was not lingering thoughts about my clinic that propelled me to write this book in the end. Instead, it was my experiences outside of the clinic, with my children, husband, and acquaintances that convinced me I must.

I followed my eldest daughter as she traveled around the country for her musical theater career. On college campuses, in Busch Gardens, in New York City, and on a Disney cruise ship, I heard her sing and act her heart out to my absolute delight. At the same time, I witnessed many of her musical theater colleagues, male and female alike, struggling with body image and weight management issues—issues that held the tremendous power to either derail or accelerate their careers. These individuals suffered in silence; they never considered seeking help for the disordered eating behavior that was a normal part of their chosen industry.

I watched my son struggle to climb the ladder toward a career in medicine, surviving twenty-four-hour shifts on minimal sleep, coffee, and a few handfuls of gummy bears. As I spoke to him about his own health-care needs, I was shocked to learn just how lacking nutritional education in medical schools remains today. It reminded me of my own medical school education on these topics thirty years ago. My husband, a cardiac surgeon, shares this feeling; even today, he comes to me for advice on how to advise his patients to optimize their health through their diets.

It was in my seven years as a 'Dance Mom,' however, that I found my most compelling reason to write. My youngest daughter, Ileana, attended two ballet boarding schools and danced professionally until an injury made her change career plans. Throughout her time in this incredibly demanding and competitive world, I helped Ileana tackle complex issues like athlete nutrition, disordered eating, and excessive exercise, not just for herself, but for her friends, colleagues, and role models as well. The stories of countless individuals, imprisoned by disordered eating and weight-related issues, appeared to me as a cry for help, and ideas for this book percolated constantly.

Between my visits and conversations with my children, I received calls from friends and family members about loved ones, from every walk of life, who were also struggling with disordered eating, whether they knew it to be that or not. I watched people all around me slip in and out of one fad diet after another. I saw friends and acquaintances endure huge weight swings. Everywhere I went, people were eager to share their stories, eager for help, and eager for a weight management plan that would not leave them starved and weak.

As I said, I have never considered myself a writer. But my daughter, Ileana, loves to write. I can honestly say that without her collaboration, this book would not exist. Together, we have written and rewritten various versions of this book. Together, we outline plans for proactively tackling problems with body image, disordered eating, obesity, dieting, and all their associated health complications.

Some people might think that writing a book that addresses eating disorders and obesity together is antithetical or that the topics are un-related. Others may argue that this approach is overly ambitious since confronting each issue is overwhelming in its own right.

In my opinion, there is no other way to tackle these issues except in tandem. Eating disorders and obesity are highly connected by underlying psychological baggage, social stigma, and medical consequences. What's more, these illnesses are symptoms of our society's failed dietary practices and decades of nutritional misinformation. Thus, knowledge about what works, what doesn't work, and why is crucial to recovery from every manifestation of these eating-related problems, be it anorexia, binge-eating disorder, bulimia, obesity, or unspecified disordered eating behavior. In every case, the victim's injured metabolism needs to be resuscitated through the establishment of long-term healthy lifestyle practices, not just temporary quick fixes.

Yes, this book is far-reaching. It needs to be. The solution must be as comprehensive as the problem is pervasive, and if we look around, we can see that this problem has indeed become disastrously pervasive.

Obesity-related diseases are literally killing our society. They create and contribute to most of our major illnesses, such as type-2 diabetes, high blood pressure, strokes, heart attacks, heart failure, cancer, gallstones, below-the-waist degenerative osteoarthritis, sleep apnea, gout, and metabolic syndrome. All of these diseases rob individuals of both their quality and quantity of life, and moreover, they place a huge burden on everyone involved in the cycle of their care: family members, employers, taxpayers, insurance carriers, health-care providers, and the government.

In 2015, the State of Obesity estimated that America spends roughly 210 billion dollars, or about 24 percent of the nation's total medical budget, on obesity related health problems.[1] Worse yet, the 2016 obesity statistics reveal how ineffective our so-called *War on Obesity* has been: In fact, the problem has reached an all-time high with 38% of adults and 17% of teenagers meeting the criteria for obesity.[2] Unless something is done to reverse this momentum, millions of individual victims and our nation as a whole are doomed to carry the weight of a crippling health catastrophe.

The introduction to this book, "A Disordered Eating Society," more fully dissects the statistics on obesity and examines the connection between this epidemic and our extremely high rate of disordered eating. By dispelling the idea that these topics are unrelated—a dangerous misconception that impedes our society's ability to recover—I advocate for the health of every reader, no matter where he or she falls on the disordered eating spectrum (including those health-conscious readers who fall safely in the middle).

My hope for my readers is that they will experience the joy of living a life free from diets, expensive weight-loss products, grueling workout regimens, weight management fears, and psychological shame. I want to steer them away from the patterns that lead to metabolic failure or ill health and guide them into lifelong patterns that create a stable, healthy, and lean future. When the knowledge of nutritional science is our road map for eating and the practice of cognitive therapy is our daily bread, this future is attainable. With this book, I aim to empower my readers with the intellectual and psychological tools necessary to realize the healthy, satiated, and abundant life.

Ileana Riverón

My mom and I sometimes joke that, in me, she's created a Frankenstein. Everything Dr. Heidi Wohlrabe learned in her training—everything she put in this book—was part of my upbringing. While other kids grew up on SpaghettiO's, Fruit Roll-Ups, and chicken nuggets, I grew up on a colorful diet of fresh produce, nuts, cheese, avocados, and lean protein sources. Even more important, I understood the reasons why, because my mom fed me with not just nutritious food but also nutritional education. And Goody-Two-shoes little me followed this knowledge to a T.

By our society's standards, my pipsqueak self was a freak of nature for loving broccoli and hating popsicles and for knowing that counting calories is idiocy but having an understanding of the glycemic index is important. I certainly don't blame people for finding my quirkiness amusing and frankly, a bit absurd. Yet when I became a preprofessional and later professional ballet dancer, my unusual upbringing became one of my greatest assets.

While dancing at the Harid Conservatory, the Royal Ballet School, and the Boston Ballet, I was able to eat more than 2,300 calories per day, almost double what some women eat, and still maintain the desired ballerina figure. Logically, most people attributed this to my physically demanding career. But that wasn't the reason. After all, many of my fellow dancers ate far fewer calories than I did and put themselves through grueling workouts in addition to our daily rehearsal schedule, yet still struggled constantly with being told they were too heavy. Nevertheless, even I couldn't shake the idea that the only reason for my good fortune was the athletic nature of my profession. After I stopped dancing professionally, I kept waiting in fear for the inevitable weight gain, as if my body was going to spontaneously balloon up and carry me into the sky with its newfound phantasmic buoyancy. I am relieved to say that no such thing has happened to date.

The real reason that I never fell prey to an eating disorder or to the terrible cycle of insecurity and shame, calorie restriction, reactionary bingeing, and then more shame and calorie restriction was because of what my mom had taught me and how she had presented it. Instead of giving me a list of oversimplified dos and don'ts, like most diet resources do, she taught me the biology of how food breaks down in the body. Equipped with this knowledge, I was able to build my own meals and snacks around scientific principles and the understanding of what my instrument (my body) needed to optimize stamina, strength, and satisfaction. And the best part? I grew up learning that healthy food was delicious and life-giving—a beautiful thing, not a negative thing. Eating healthily was never something I needed to *impose* on myself. As a result, I never felt restricted by rules, and I never had anything to rebel against through bingeing.

When I left my ballet career and entered Harvard College, I was surprised and dismayed to realize that body image issues, disordered eating, and dieting are not just a ballerina problem; they are prevalent among people of every body type and from every socioeconomic and cultural background. This sad realization reinforced my gratitude toward my mom for giving me the tools necessary for lifelong physical and psychological health. Odd as it may sound, I am immensely thankful to be her greatest test case, her Frankenstein.

Since my life is in many ways a testimony to the effectiveness of what Dr. Wohlrabe teaches, I am happy to have had the opportunity to coauthor her book. Over the past six years, Dr. Wohlrabe put into writing her expertise as a psychiatrist and eating disorders specialist, and I helped her research, edit, and rewrite the material so that it is user-friendly and entertaining. Adding funny (at least in my mind) side notes and references to *South Park*, *Mean Girls*, Harry Potter, and (keepin' it classy) Aristotle made my job a pretty sweet gig. Perhaps I got carried away at times, but I'll let you be the judge of that.

Dearest Reader, I want to end by telling you some really good news: it *is* possible. It's entirely possible to have a positive relationship with food and with your body—one that is free of shame or obsessiveness—to enjoy meals that are as delicious as they are nutritious, to feel satiated but not guilty, to eat healthily on a budget, to be active and fit without torturous workouts, and to be thin as well as strong and full of energy. Whether you're a ballerina, a student, an overworked mom or dad, an athlete, an academician, you name it, this kind of life is absolutely within your grasp. Don't sell yourself short. You are more than worth it.

~ 1 ~

A Disordered Eating Society

Our society is fixated on diet, body shape, and exercise. And yet, despite our obsessions, weight-related health issues continue to spiral out of control, including hypertension, diabetes, and all forms of eating disorders. The shocking statistics tell the tale all too well. In the early 1980s—not very long ago at all—very few of our children were struggling with obesity or eating disorders. Only 4 percent of children in the United States were overweight.[1] Today, we've reached an all time high; 33 percent of children are considered overweight and 17 percent obese![2] Continuing on this trend, *half* of the next generation's children will be overweight—a prediction that illuminates the dire future we have set up for this nation's health.

The rate of eating disorders has followed a parallel pattern. In the seventies and eighties, public awareness was just starting to grow regarding this rare but dangerous group of illnesses. Today, as many as twenty-four million Americans suffer from an eating disorder, 95 percent of whom are between the ages of twelve and twenty-five years old.[3,4]

I don't know about you, but these statistics break my heart. They show that a terrible change has taken place in the last thirty years: obesity and eating disorders have gone from being the rare exception to widespread epidemics. And their concurrent upsurge is not a coincidence. The rise of eating disorders is absolutely linked to the onset of the obesity crisis.

So what are we doing wrong? We certainly do not suffer from a shortage of resources. After all, diet books fill the shelves of bookstores everywhere, just as health-food products line the shelves of every grocery store. Still, as the amount of available information has grown exponentially over the past few decades, so too have our food-related disorders and diseases.

The horrifying truth is this: We have a runaway weight and eating crisis that, so far, no one has been able to stop. It is high time that we figure out how to turn these statistics around. That's why I'm here: to give you the skinny on how to be lean and healthy for life. I'm not saying it's going to be easy. Our widespread disordered eating problem cannot be solved by simply telling people to watch their diets and exercise. If it could, we would have averted this crisis long ago.

I propose that we take a three-step approach to tackling this issue. First, we need to grasp the nature of the problem. Let's figure out the hows, whys, whens, and whos of this epidemic. Second, we need to learn about the science of metabolism and uncover important research about how our bodies use food. Let's weed through all of the contradicting nutritional advice out there and figure out exactly what is fact and what is fiction. Last, but certainly not least, we need to assemble all of the psychological tools necessary for insight and change. By the end of this book, you're going to be an expert on what works, what doesn't work, and why. My hope is that together, we can make healthy living a practical and satisfying option for you.

What Happened?
What Are the Origins of the Weight Problem?

I hate to admit it, but the responsibility for the current weight crisis falls largely on the shoulders of the parents of this current generation—the baby boomers. We might have had the best of intentions, but the truth is, we fed our kids the wrong food as toddlers, we overfed them as they grew up, and worst of all, whether we realized it or not, we fed them the wrong information about nutrition all along the way.

Picture this typical scenario. A young mother decides to introduce green beans into her baby's diet for the first time. Mom puts a spoonful of green mush into little Timmy's mouth. Within seconds, the green beans are hurled into the air and sprayed all over Mom's clean white shirt. She watches in frustration as her distressed toddler wrinkles his nose and shakes his head, refusing another bite. Nothing more will pass between those two little pouty lips. After ten minutes of struggle, the green beans appear to be everywhere *except* in baby Timmy's stomach. Timmy's mom quickly becomes fed up. Meanwhile, little Timmy is still hungry. In quiet resignation, Mom pulls out a cereal box. She easily gets Timmy to eat cereal, snarf down peaches, and gum up cookies.

So who taught whom what? The only one who learned anything from this experience was Mom. She learned that in order to get food into little Timmy's stomach, she must cater to Timmy's taste buds.

This is not an unusual scene in today's world. We parents know that toddlers become quiet in church or at a restaurant with a cracker, cookie, or juice box. Mom can buy herself a few seconds of peace by giving little Timmy some type of simple carbohydrate to nibble on. Foods my generation was taught to appreciate growing up, like broccoli, mushrooms, and asparagus, have been replaced by kids' meals. You know what I mean—those nutrient-poor, ketchup- or syrup-laden, carbohydrate conglomerations that we serve our children three times daily.

Let's look at a typical meal plan for a young child in the United States.

> Breakfast: 2 Pop-Tarts and a glass of orange juice (more than 90 percent of the calories come from simple, refined carbohydrates)
>
> Lunch: 1.5 cups of macaroni and cheese, ½ cup of applesauce, ½ cup of corn and peas medley, and a glass of chocolate milk (nearly all of the calories come from refined or simple carbohydrates)
>
> Snack: fruit snacks and chips (again, refined or simple carbs)
>
> Dinner: chicken fingers, mashed potatoes, skim milk, and a few green beans (While this is a little healthier, there is still little fiber and the majority of the calories are still carbs and some fat.)
>
> Dessert: chocolate-chip cookie with ice cream (Need I say more?)
>
> Summary of the day's calories: 90 percent carbohydrates

If you want to pinpoint a leading cause for the obesity crisis, this is it. Carbohydrates are the staples for breakfast, lunch, dinner, and snacks. According to the *Journal of the American Dietetic Association*, 40 percent of the total calories in two- to eighteen-year-olds' diets come from empty calories provided by sugary drinks, desserts, and pizza.[5]

Nutritionally, kids' meals are not a decent replacement for a balanced, home-cooked meal. But my goodness are they ever convenient and easy! And convenience and ease rule in this fast-paced world. We just don't have the time to prepare fresh food anymore. Lucky for us, modern science has figured out how to save us the time it takes to prepare food. Dry, sweet, simple carbohydrates packaged in airtight containers can be transported everywhere and anywhere with minimal mess and effort and no worry of spoilage. Three years later, the chemically preserved cuisine is as good as ever. It's a miracle!

Another handy invention for busy parents trying to feed their families on a budget is the fast-food restaurant, the number of which has more than doubled since the 1970s.[6] While driving home from work, Mom or Dad can swing by the drive-through window at McDonald's and pick up burgers, fries, and shakes without even leaving the car. Children can eat while driving across town and still make it to soccer practice or piano lessons on time. And much to a parent's delight, dinner comes complaint-free. Forget about nasty-tasting broccoli and asparagus. Kids can get their daily requirement of vitamins and minerals through a serving of ketchup!

Having grown up on it, our population loves cheap, starchy, highly palatable food. So manufacturers pander to our cravings, smiling all the way to the bank. They gladly refine carbohydrates, strip them of fiber, add sweeteners, and package them so they last until Armageddon. And when the public becomes tolerant of this sweetness, what happens then? What do the manufacturers do when their products don't seem as deliciously addicting anymore? Easy. They sit in their tall black swivel chairs and let out their best evil laugh—before they pour more cheap, concentrated corn syrup into their food, making it sweeter than ever before!

Okay, so they're not all evil, cape-wearing villains. But you get the picture, right? America's exaggerated sweet tooth is the reason we find corn syrup at the top of the ingredients lists of most manufactured foods: sauces, condiments, salad dressings, canned goods, packaged items, beverages, and so on.

Not only has the trans-fat-rich, sugar-loaded, corn-syrup-soaked diet become a part of everyday life; it has become inextricably linked to the celebration of all of life's major milestones. Think about it; food remains the central theme for most special events. Birthdays, anniversaries, Christmas, Easter, Valentine's Day, Halloween, and Thanksgiving would not feel right without their respective confections. Besides, can you think of a better way to celebrate a victory or mourn a loss than through an ice cream sundae? Let's see ... Your boyfriend dumped you? Here's a box of chocolates. It's our anniversary? Here's a box of chocolates. Hard day at work? Here's a box of chocolates. Your hamster just died? ... Well, do you like chocolate?

Food is like magic. It can fill awkward silences, mark special occasions, heal pain, cement bonds of friendship, and reward hard work. If we were to try to break up the emotional connections between food and comfort, love, and celebration, well, that would just be heartless. We might as well start practicing our evil laughs and invest in our very own tall swivel chairs and black capes.

Taking all of this into consideration, it's obvious that the kids'-meal-championing baby boomer parents aren't the only ones to blame. The food industry, as well as unhealthy social conventions, have done just as much to dig us into this mess. Actually, in many cases, the parents are equal parts victim and perpetrator, for adults and kids alike have fallen prey to incorrect and misguiding nutritional information. For years, the public has been misled and misfed. We weren't given the right facts about how food is biologically used by the body. We were never told how to improve metabolism. Basically, we were never taught how to stay thin and healthy.

Do you remember the old food pyramid that, for decades, was supposed to be our guide to nutritional health? I do. I spent years running an eating disorders clinic, working with dietitians who followed this food pyramid as if it were the law. The only problem (and what a huge problem it is) was that it inevitably put weight on each of our normal or already overweight patients. As a result, I had a major predicament on my hands: how could I keep the trust of my patients if they put on weight while working with our dietitians?[7]

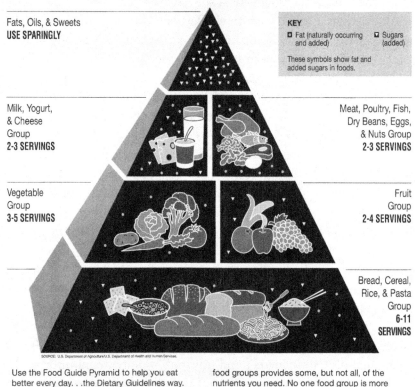

Food Guide Pyramid

A Guide to Daily Food Choices

Fats, Oils, & Sweets
USE SPARINGLY

KEY
◻ Fat (naturally occurring ☐ Sugars
and added) (added)

These symbols show fat and
added sugars in foods.

Milk, Yogurt,
& Cheese
Group
2-3 SERVINGS

Meat, Poultry, Fish,
Dry Beans, Eggs,
& Nuts Group
2-3 SERVINGS

Vegetable
Group
3-5 SERVINGS

Fruit
Group
2-4 SERVINGS

Bread, Cereal,
Rice, & Pasta
Group
6-11
SERVINGS

SOURCE: U.S. Department of Agriculture/U.S. Department of Health and Human Services.

Use the Food Guide Pyramid to help you eat better every day. . .the Dietary Guidelines way. Start with plenty of Breads, Cereals, Rice, and Pasta; Vegetables; and Fruits. Add two to three servings from the Milk group and two to three servings from the Meat group. Each of these food groups provides some, but not all, of the nutrients you need. No one food group is more important than another — for good health you need them all. Go easy on fats, oils, and sweets, the foods in the small tip of the Pyramid.

US Department of Agriculture

The emphasis of the old food pyramid was to cut the intake of fats. But wait a minute. Isn't that still the emphasis? What's wrong with that? Well, nothing—except that a person will inevitably gain weight when the vast majority of his or her calories come from refined grains and simple sugars. It's as predictable as the fate of a one-armed trapeze artist.

The fact that we've been digesting incorrect information about something as vital as health is especially astonishing when you consider the high-tech age in which we live. We have unbelievable access to a world of information, right at our fingertips! Yet this fast-paced age of technology has failed to equip us with accurate knowledge about nutrition. It has, however, provided us with a very different kind of skill: we are all expert multitaskers. Kids can surf the Internet, text, and change TV channels while doing their homework. Adults can check e-mail or play Sudoku on their phones while sitting in a meeting or watching a soccer game. Having grown accustomed to this constant stream of intense stimulation, it's no wonder that no one wants to tediously slice the tops off of fresh green beans or watch a soup simmer for two hours.

This is the world our children are growing up in. And it is different, so very different, from the way things have been historically.

Let's think about this for a second. There were far fewer obese people one hundred years ago. Why is that? Why are clothes in vintage shops or in museums so very tiny? How did people eat complete meals and never struggle with obesity back then?

Throughout history, food accumulation, preparation, and consumption occupied a significant portion of a family's time and energy. This profound focus on food was necessary for survival and was driven by both biological need and cultural cues. And this wasn't only characteristic of the Dark Ages. On the contrary, it held true until relatively recently. Even if we were to look back one or two generations, the world of consumption would be almost unrecognizable to us now.

When my mother was growing up, it was common for people to have gardens and to enjoy the bounty of their produce all through the summer and fall. Any excess produce was canned and kept in storage. With good weather conditions, it was possible to can enough to feed a family of eight through the winter and spring months.

I can't imagine the amount of work that was spent weeding, gathering, and canning for a family of that size. Everyone, from the oldest to the youngest, worked hard to contribute. Space was limited in iceboxes and was therefore reserved for dairy products and meat storage.

Cabinets contained canned goods and baking goods. There was little that was readily available for snacking. So if you were hungry, you had to really spend time preparing food. What a foreign concept that is to us now! No bags of chips or boxes of cookies to grab on the go!

But this isn't a pity fest for the people of the past. Because they took such care in cooking and baking, most of their food was phenomenal. I vividly remember my grandmother's egg pancakes; they were some of the most delicious things I have ever tasted in my life. And I'll never forget eating her homemade ice cream and thinking I was in heaven. But nothing was edible without effort.

Today, our kitchen cabinets are packed with chocolate-chip cookies, marshmallows, crackers, chips, and so many other delicious, ready-to-eat snacks. Hmmm, could this be our problem?

It's not that food is less of a focal point in our lives today than it was historically. But instead of going into cultivating, harvesting, preserving, and preparing, all of our energy goes into one of two things: either quick and easy consumption or the attempt *not* to consume. That's what's new. The struggle to restrain ourselves from eating, as a widespread social phenomenon, is a fad of our current era. According to the American Dietetic Association, "46% of 9–11 year olds are 'sometimes' or 'very often' on diets, and 82% of their families are 'sometimes' or 'very often' on diets."[8] Dieting is a fight against one's most basic instincts, a way of training oneself to ignore biological cues. It fosters a fear of food that is unnatural, counterinstinctual, and in the end, counterproductive, for it puts us on the fast track to the very pathologic eating behavior that leads to eating disorders. Thus, it's sad to say, but when it comes to nutrition, evolutionary changes have been destructive rather than advantageous. The *progress* that has allowed us to forego hunting, gathering, and preparing food has led to the downfall of health.

Do you really think that we were mistakenly programmed to become overweight if we ate according to our hunger? I think not. Is it the natural course of life for us to be poisoning ourselves with pollution? Erm ... not so much. I think that we have ignorantly luxuriated in our brilliant conveniences to the point of a health crisis. We have stripped the original food from God's garden of much of its nutritional value by removing the fiber that aids in satiety and nutrition. Then we serve this white, sweet, pasty clump of fakeness to our children in many different forms throughout the day.

We are overfed but undernourished. Though we should be able to easily and comfortably eat the healthy produce of our land, in truth, we look more like an obese society living in a nutritional wasteland. It's no wonder that our nutritional deficits and fear of food have spawned a slew of pathologic and disordered eating behaviors.

But here's the good news. The human body can still improve and thrive if one makes the right changes. Right now, we have an incredible opportunity. We have the opportunity to slow down the obesity progression, prevent the continued rise of eating disorders, and recover our health. We can all learn so much from our mistakes, and we can all learn so much from science. So let's do just that and start our journey on the road to health.

At the end of each chapter in this book, you will find a bulleted list of the chapter's main takeaways. You can use these as a way to solidify what you've just read and as an easy reference point in the future.

Summary
A Disordered Eating Society

- Obesity and eating disorders are both trending upward, suggesting a connection between them.

- Diet products, programs, and books have done nothing to impact these trends.

- Over the past century, sociologic changes and agricultural developments have contributed to the rise of obesity and eating disorders.

  - We no longer work long hours procuring and storing organic food. Food, especially unhealthy food, is too easily and readily available to us.

  - Our fast-paced society always chooses convenience over labor. This holds true when it comes to eating, thus the popularity of fast food, prepackaged meals, prepackaged snacks, and so on.

  - The development of corn syrup has allowed for food to be sweeter than ever before. Our palates have become increasingly tolerant to sweetness, and as a result, we crave high glycemic index foods.

- By feeding our children white, pasty, high glycemic foods many times throughout the day, we fail to teach them how to eat right and set them up for a lifetime of unhealthy diets.

- The food pyramid, which promoted carbohydrates while discouraging sufficient amounts of fats, proteins, and vegetables, has only contributed to our society's eating problems.

- We are a society that is calorically overfed yet undernourished. Faulty nutritional information has repeatedly sabotaged our chances of recovering.

~ 2 ~

Dieting: The Gateway Drug

Surveys show that most Americans have, at some point in their lives, put themselves on a diet. But despite the fact that dieting is one of America's national pastimes, our country continues to struggle with weight issues. In fact, recent Centers for Disease Control (CDC) statistics indicate that roughly *two-thirds* of the adult population is currently overweight and about 36 percent is obese.[1] And the numbers continue to rise.

So here's an interesting thought: Could there be a connection between dieting behavior and weight gain?

Hmmmm ... This is something I want to explore with you. We'll start with some pertinent statistics.

- About 41 percent of Americans are on a diet at any given time, and about 63 percent of people have dieted at least once during their lifetime.[2]

- In 1986, a *Wall Street Journal* reporter interviewed one hundred fourth-grade girls in order to learn about dieting behavior in children. Surprisingly, 80 percent of them were dieting at the time of the interview. (Keep in mind that these are *fourth*-grade girls!) Then again, in 2009, twenty-three years later, this same journalist decided to contact as many of the women from the original study as he could find. Lo and behold, these grown-up, thirty-two-year-old women admitted that they were never able to escape their obsessions with weight, food, or body image.[3]

- A Canadian study found that 37 percent of girls in grade nine and 40 percent of girls in grade ten thought they were too fat. Of those who were *normal* weight (based on a normal BMI), 19 percent believed that they were too fat![4]

- More telling yet, an American study found that 51 percent of *nine- and ten-year-old* girls felt more comfortable with themselves if they were on a diet. And a whopping 81 percent of *ten-year-olds* feared being fat.[5] Again, we see the correlation between the obesity crisis, a consequent fear of food, and dieting behavior—even among elementary school children!

- Ninety-one percent of college students have dieted in order to manage their weight, and 22 percent diet "often" or "always."[6]

- Another study found that 46 percent of *nine- to eleven-year-olds* are either "sometimes" or "very often" on diets. Meanwhile, 82 percent of their family members are often on diets.[7] So it seems to run in the family. Children can pick up disordered eating from their parents and start early with their own unhealthy eating behaviors.

- Thirty-five percent of "occasional dieters" progress into pathological dieting (disordered eating), and as many as 25 percent advance to full-blown eating disorders.[8]

- From a study called Project EAT, involving nearly five thousand teens, we learn that more than 50 percent of girls and more than 33 percent of boys engage in unhealthy weight-control behaviors, such as fasting, smoking, use of diet pills, vomiting, or the use of laxatives. The higher-weight and obese teens were more likely to engage in binge-eating and unhealthy weight control tactics than the normal-weight teens.[9]

As you can see, it's not an exaggeration to dub dieting a national pastime, right up there with baseball and barbecues. Moreover, we see that being overweight, in and of itself, appears to be a risk factor for both dieting *and* disordered eating. Obesity, dieting, and eating disorders seem to go hand in hand.

Particularly heartbreaking to me is the fact that dieting behavior begins at such young ages. Fourth-grade children should be focusing on learning and playing, not how to resist their instincts to eat. I guess the problem was inevitable, however. Dieting is our treatment of choice for not only a fat body, but also a fat phobia, which is almost universal in our society.

Universal Fat Phobia and the Diet Industry

As a society, we don't like being fat, and we're uncomfortable with fat people. All too often, negative attributes are unfairly ascribed to the obese. We assume that they're lazy, unmotivated, and even unclean. We'd rather be almost anything than fat.[10] Think that's an overstatement? Then get a load of this: 30 percent of thin people would rather experience a divorce than be obese,[11] and 46 percent of thin people would rather give up a year of their lives than be obese.[12] According to a study done in 1996, 50 percent of eighteen- to twenty-five-year-old females would rather be struck by a truck than be fat![13] And two-thirds of these women would rather be stupid or mean than be fat![14]

Crazy, right? The pain we'd endure to avoid being fat is startling!

This is precisely what fuels the entire diet industry (including weight-loss programs, drugs, and surgical procedures), which are projected to rake in a staggering $315 billion in 2015.[15] Quite an extraordinary moneymaker, I must say! But the strangest thing is this: weight-loss programs don't need to provide any evidence of long-term success in order to reap big profits. They only need to sell the idea of weight loss in order to get people to fork over cash.

The dieting industry knows its target audience well. They prey off the fact that poor, ignorant dieters feel lost without them. Clients depend upon weight-loss companies for their diet food, diet books, and diet sessions. Women and men are willing to pay outrageous amounts of money for teeny tiny portions of food or simply for the *opportunity* to shed a few pounds. However, the sad truth is that this industry gains big profits by perpetuating dieting myths, not by producing results.

Skeptical? Well, see for yourself.

Researchers at UCLA examined thirty-one long-term diet studies. They found that about two-thirds of dieters regained *more* weight within four or five years than they initially lost.[16] A coauthor from this group, Janet Tomiyama, stated, "We asked 'what evidence is there that dieting works in the long term?,' and found that the evidence shows the opposite. Several studies indicate that dieting is actually a consistent predictor of future weight gain."[17]

Wow. So dieting can actually do more harm in the long run than it does good in the short run!

CBS News noted that most weight-loss programs don't share detailed outcome studies of their diet plans. And maybe you've already noticed that they never talk about long-term success. Maybe this is why: "A review of 10 of the nation's most popular weight-loss programs found that except for Weight Watchers, none of them offer proof that they actually work at helping people shed pounds and keep them off. Only Weight Watchers had strong documentation that it worked— with one study showing that participants lost around 5 percent (about 10 lbs) of their initial weight in six months and kept off about half of it two years later."[18]

Even the success of Weight Watchers is extremely *under*whelming. Keeping half of the weight off after two years? Based on this trend, what do you think happens *after* two years? And what do you think happens when these people finally leave the program? Judging from other programs' statistics, my Magic 8 Ball says, "Outlook not so good."

Expensive commercial diet programs aren't the only diets that fail; they all do. "Ninety-five percent of diets fail and most will regain their lost weight in 1–5 years," says the Council on Size and Weight Discrimination.[19] And just to put a nail in the coffin, here's one more fact: Adolescent girls who diet are at 324 percent greater risk for obesity than those who do not diet.[20] Did you get that?

Pause. Rewind. Read that last statement one more time. Let it sink in …

Okay, play. Diets don't work in the long run.

Reasons for Diet Failures

When diets fail, we tend to blame the dieters. We think to ourselves, *They didn't try hard enough. They obviously just lacked willpower* (as we flip our hair over our shoulders and stick our noses in the air). But what if there are good reasons why diets fail?

Okay, you're about to have a gazillion questions thrown at you. You'll probably want to glaze over like a Krispy Kreme doughnut and move on. But please resist that urge and think about these questions in your head.

- What types of diets have you tried?
- How long were you able to stay on any particular diet?
- Were you consistent in following it?
- How did you feel while on the diet? Any fatigue, irritability, or excessive hunger? Okay …
- Why did you stop the diet?
- Would you say it worked?
- How long did you keep the weight off?
- Did you go gain more weight after easing up on the food restrictions?

If you have dieted, you most likely have personal experience with how frustrating it is. Odds are that you have returned to your previous weight, perhaps with a few extra pounds for good measure too.

Let's begin examining the reasons for dieting failures.

First of all, when people diet, they neglect their own body's hunger cues. Instead of responding to the brain's cravings or the gut's hunger, they begin to rely on conscious mental cues to rule their eating behavior. For example, at lunch, a craving for a grilled-cheese-and-ham sandwich is ignored in favor of a low-fat, low-salt, low-protein pasta/lettuce salad. When the conscientious restricters fail to feel satiated, they may find themselves obsessing over food, nibbling on all sorts of needless things that do not supply the protein, salt, or fat that their body was craving.

Ignoring body cues like this interrupts neurohormonal systems that control hunger, satiety, weight regulation, sleep, energy levels, and mood. The poor body becomes confused and messed up. It stops knowing what to feel when.

As if that weren't bad enough, starvation causes the brain to continuously obsess over food. People develop "hungry eyes" with restrictive eating. Their hunger builds and builds but is suppressed time and time again, until finally those big, hungry eyes want to eat everything in sight. When the dieters are alone in the kitchen at night and vulnerable from fatigue, tasting just one cookie doesn't seem to cut this hunger. A box of cookies does. Guilt doesn't linger far behind. Understandably, the dieters are torn up over their failure. They may search for some way to erase their gluttonous mistake. Purging, whether through vomiting, exercising, or laxative use, seems like a way to undo destructive over-eating. Before long, people find themselves involved in typical bulimic patterns: hunger, binge, guilt, purge, hunger. It's a terrible, vicious cycle.

That's how dieting can lead directly into disordered eating patterns. Remember the fact presented earlier? Just in case, here it is again: 35 percent of normal dieters get involved in disordered, pathological eating behaviors. And of those 35 percent, roughly one-fourth become eating disordered.[21]

I'm sorry to be such a Debbie Downer, but it gets even worse ...

Dieting not only sets people up for disordered eating, but it also prevents future weight loss. Yeah, that's right—it makes it *harder* for you to lose weight the next time you decide to diet. Great. As if losing weight weren't hard enough already!

Dieting triggers a defensive maneuver by the body—in essence, a sit-down strike. This amazing defensive move not only prevents you from reaching your goal today; it also moves that goal further and further out of your reach the more you continue to diet.

Exactly how does your body do this self-defeating maneuver?

Essentially, a Chernobyl type of nuclear meltdown occurs. The body's response to a decrease in caloric intake is to *shut down*. Basically, when calories are restricted, our bodies expend less energy in order to keep us alive. God gifted us with this adaptive mechanism to help our species survive during prolonged famines.

The meltdown is rather subtle at first. The body gets colder, slows down its production of oils, and slows down the heart rate. Lethargy, crabbiness, and fatigue are common as the lights are dimmed throughout the body. As people lose more weight, this protective mechanism becomes even more exaggerated. Over time, more and more body systems fail.

Because of the progressive nature of the meltdown, once you start losing weight on a particular diet, it gets harder and harder to lose the same amounts of weight, even if you maintain your same dieting patterns. As a result, you will need to restrict calories even further to continue losing weight or even to maintain your new weight! An ever-decreasing number of calories becomes essential for weight loss. Like the Greek myth of Sisyphus rolling the boulder up a mountain for all eternity, dieters are faced with a never-ending, uphill battle. And as they go, the incline only gets steeper.

If the weight loss is quick—more than one to two pounds per week—lean body tissue or muscle will be lost in addition to fat. To those of you who feel you have too much bulky muscle, this might not sound too bad. But losing muscle further reduces your metabolism, perpetuating the problem even more. So although every overweight individual wants to see the pounds melt right off as if with a blowtorch, that is not a healthy goal. In fact, it's counterproductive—that is, if you want to stay thin for decades rather than just months.

If all this information is not enough to frighten you, here are a few more interesting tidbits.

Some studies indicate that repeated patterns of dieting actually lead to a resistance toward weight loss. Hence, it takes *longer* to lose the *same amount* of weight on *fewer* calories with *each* successive cycle.

A study (done by psychologist Kelly Brownwell and his colleagues from the University of Pennsylvania School of Medicine) described what happened to rats that were subjected to yo-yo dieting, or on-and-off restrictive eating patterns. In the first round of dieting, it took twenty-one days for the rats to lose a small amount of weight. But in the second round of dieting, it took *forty-six days* to lose that same amount of weight! That's more than twice as long! In addition, the rats put the weight back on each time *in successively shorter periods*. Whereas it took a full forty-six days to gain the weight back after the first round, it only took fourteen days after the second round.[22]

Ugh. How miserable is that?

An older study, done in 1978, proved that starved animals gain weight at a much quicker rate than animals that had never been on a restrictive diet before. Researchers Peter Boyle, Leonard Storlien, and Richard Keesey found that rats who were starved to 20 percent below their original weight gained 29.6 grams while the nonstarved rats gained only 1.6 grams on the same type of food. Importantly, the starved rats were eating somewhat *less* than the nonstarved rats, and they still regained the weight faster![23]

What conclusions can we make from these studies? It seems that our bodies get better at maintaining weight and storing fat with each recurrent episode of dieting. Think about how absolutely frustrating that is for all those well-intended dieters. Perhaps they actually have the willpower to diet but give up when they experience this phenomenon over and over again. And who can blame them? Starving yourself is miserable, but gaining weight despite it all? That's just plain awful.

Psychological Issues Associated with Dieting

The process of dieting leads to all sorts of strange, self-defeating thinking patterns. For example, a dieter anticipating a new diet might tell him- or herself, "This is my last chance to pig out. I'm gonna let myself have one major splurge before the fasting begins." With that, the person consumes large quantities of highly caloric food the night before the diet begins, making the task at hand even more difficult and overwhelming than it was originally.

Self-defeating thinking patterns like this lead to self-defeating behavior. This fact was proven in a recent study, reported by the *Journal of Social and Clinical Psychology*, which involved two groups of college-age females: one group of dieters and one of non-dieters. Before the study even began, all participants were offered 1, 2, or 3 milkshakes, and then they entered into what appeared to be an ice cream taste test. Basically, the researchers created and then observed an all-you-can-eat ice cream extravaganza. Among the dieters, a puzzling trend emerged: the more milkshakes a participant had consumed before the study began, the *more* ice cream she went on to eat during the taste test. The non-dieters, on the other hand, acted in a more rational way. The more milkshakes a non-dieter had consumed prior to the study, the *less* ice cream she went on to eat during the taste test.[24, 25]

How does that make sense? Why would the dieting participants who'd eaten the greatest amount of fattening food beforehand go on to eat the most ice cream during the taste test?

This baffling phenomenon takes place because of the dieter's pathologic thinking: *I already blew my diet so why not go all out?* The non-dieters in the ice cream study didn't have these kinds of thoughts, so they had less trouble controlling how much junk food they ate.

Most people have given in to this *letting loose* behavior at some point, but just think about how mistaken this line of thinking is! If you have one cookie and you blew your diet, having five more *does* matter! Bingeing with one brownie is *not* the same as bingeing with four brownies. Don't fall prey to this all-or-nothing thinking.

Unfortunately, there's more. For instance, dieters are also more prone to emotional/stress eating than non-dieters. Similarly, they are more prone to unconscious/automatic eating when their minds are preoccupied. Picture this: Sandy Smith is a dieter. She comes home, exhausted after a long day, and turns on her favorite TV show. She's distracted. Her guard is down. (I can almost hear the scary movie music in the background.) If Sandy weren't a dieter, her hand would be less likely to continue moving from the bowl of popcorn to her mouth. But since she is a dieter and her body is starved, she is extremely vulnerable to unconscious or emotional eating. Sandy Smith has been sabotaged by her own body's desire to put fat back on. Anytime attention is diverted from the extraordinary self-control it takes to starve oneself, a dieter can consume way too many calories.[26]

I know this is a research-heavy chapter, and I'm sorry to throw so many studies at you, but you can't miss this one. Ancel Keyes and his colleagues at the University of Minnesota conducted a landmark study in 1950 that would never be allowed today—for a lot of reasons. I will try to highlight his findings, but you might want to read further about his experiments in the book *The Great Starvation Experiment: Ancel Keyes and the Men Who Starved for Science* by Todd Tucker.[27] This study reaped volumes of helpful information about the process of starvation and the dangers of dieting. It will help you understand that the symptoms we associate with anorexia and bulimia are essentially the same symptoms that can be seen with any restrictive dieting.

In 1950, one hundred healthy men were allowed to volunteer to participate in a study as an alternative to military service. The team of researchers then carefully selected thirty-six of these men whom they considered to be physically and psychologically stable and who did not have prior issues with an eating disorder or weight management.

For three months, the volunteers were observed as they ate normally. Their personalities and eating behaviors were documented as they continued with their usual eating practices and activities. Then, over the ensuing six months, the men were put on a restrictive diet that replaced only *half of their normal caloric intake*. For many of the men, that meant being put on about 1,500 calories per day. Think about that for a minute: 1,500 calories per day is typical for dieters. In fact, many people consume that amount on a daily basis for maintenance. Actually, it's not uncommon for dieters to aim for less than 1,200 calories per day. So that should give us some perspective.

On average, the men lost 25 percent of their normal weight. But I'd say the loss of personality and normal thinking patterns was even greater.

Over the period of weight loss, these men developed an extreme preoccupation with food. They talked about food, thought about it all the time, and even dreamed about food. Their interest in sex and other activities dropped significantly. Their food preoccupations included gum chewing, unusual food rituals, and very slow eating behaviors. They pored over cookbooks, enjoyed watching people eat, and found that their ability to concentrate was markedly impaired. One man rummaged through garbage cans for food. Many began hoarding food or began collecting odd items. Once the study was concluded, several men even switched occupations in order to be in food-related fields.

Consumption of coffee and tea needed to be limited to no more than nine cups per day because of the excessive intake of these liquids. Gum chewing needed to be limited as well, since one man was chomping through forty packs of gum per day. (Can you imagine the jaw aches?)

The subjects tolerated this restriction to varying degrees. Some of the subjects had several binge-eating episodes followed by terrible remorse and shame. For example, one man, while working at a grocery store, ate numerous cookies, a bag of popcorn, and several bananas before being able to stop himself. He felt nauseated and lost his cookies (quite literally) when he returned to the lab. One man needed to be released from the study because of too many episodes of loss of control, overeating, and sickness.

Through the six months of semistarvation, the volunteers complained of gastrointestinal discomfort, weakness, poor motor control, dizziness, headaches, insomnia, edema (fluid retention), hair loss, decreased tolerance for cold, hypersensitivity to noise and light, irritability, visual problems (inability to focus, eye aches, or visual spots), auditory disturbances (like ringing in the ears), and unusual feelings in the extremities, such as numbness or tingling. Wow. That sounds like the end of a drug commercial. Restricting calories caused all those side effects? Yuck.

Once the six months were over, the subjects began a twelve-week refeeding period. During this time, even though the caloric intake increased substantially, there was the same preoccupation with thoughts of food, preparation of food, binging, vomiting, shame, and self-criticism that existed during caloric restriction. The men complained of hunger immediately following a large meal. It was as if they could not be satiated.

Over the weekends, the men found it even more difficult to eat in moderation. Some men were eating between 8,000 and 10,000 calories per day, stuffing themselves to the brim and becoming ill but still feeling hungry or preoccupied with thoughts of food. It took five months for the majority of the men to regulate their eating behavior.

As we saw with the rats in the studies we discussed earlier, dieters tend to eventually gain more weight back than they lost on their diets. Ancel Keyes's men confirmed this finding too: the majority of them overshot their entrance weight by about 10 percent when they were allowed to refeed. And the worst part is, most of their regained weight came back as fat, not muscle. So not only did they weigh more than they did before they dieted, but more of their weight was from fat than before. To be specific, body fat composition increased 140 percent over their entry-level value. This highlights another ingenious defense mechanism: our bodies store up extra fat following a period of starvation just in case there's another famine coming.

Remember how the subjects chosen were the most psychologically stable of the original one hundred volunteers? Well, that's what makes this next part so disturbing. The men were plagued with emotional instability, obsessive-compulsive traits, depression, anger outbursts, anxiety, apathy, and neglect of hygiene. Several men even suffered with psychotic-type episodes.

As for their personalities, these generally outgoing, competent men became shy, withdrawn, and humorless. They struggled with feelings of inadequacy. Their interest in sex was minimal to nonexistent. And they complained of having problems with concentration, memory, and judgment.

Can you see why this study would never be allowed today? These men were almost ruined—physically, psychologically, and emotionally.

But it was so powerful in the horrific truths it revealed about restrictive eating and dieting.

Perhaps the scariest part is that people seem to change as they diet. Dieting can turn a sane person into someone who is totally irrational. You may say that you could never be anorexic or bulimic, but that's what anorexic and bulimic patients would have said too.

My daughter, a self-proclaimed Harry Potter geek, pointed out to me that dieting is like the maze in *Harry Potter and the Goblet of Fire*, and while I've never read the books myself, I think she's right. She told me that just before the contestants of the Triwizard Tournament go into their final challenge, Dumbledore warns them, "People change in the maze. Oh, find the cup if you can. But be very wary; you could just lose yourselves along the way." Once in the maze, the contestants— Harry, Cedric, Fleur, and Victor—find themselves thinking and acting in a way they never would have before the competition. It brought out hideous things in them.[28]

Restrictive eaters can reach a tipping point that launches them into their very own Triwizard Tournament maze, and suddenly, they're pushed over the precipice into the void of uncharacteristic thoughts and actions. That is how normal people can end up with a serious disease like anorexia nervosa or bulimia.[29, 30]

Don't fool yourself into thinking that you're safe, that you're too smart to fall into the trap. The eating disorder spider web is ready to catch any and all innocent dieters when they least expect it.

So why would anyone diet? The consequences are simply horrendous! And yet, think about how many people are currently suffering with the symptoms of semistarvation due to crazy dieting behavior. Think about all the women who frequently consume as few as 1,200 calories per day. Surely they just don't know that a dramatic reduction in calories paves the way for the horrific signs and symptoms of starvation to emerge, not to mention a future of even greater weight struggles than they had before.

A healthy weight loss occurs when the body is not aware that it's taking in too few calories. It occurs with normal but healthy eating and the reduction of simple carbohydrates. A subtle drop of one to two pounds per month is imperceptible to the body, and is therefore the kind of weight loss that can be sustained. Slow and steady weight loss allows your brain to still function and your mood to stay elevated, and it won't cause your body to shut down by staging a metabolic sit-down strike.

Summary
Dieting: The Gateway Drug

- Dieting ...

  - is a national pastime; roughly 41 percent of people in America are currently dieting
  - is actually a *predictor* for future weight gain
  - ruins the metabolism and sets up a resistance to weight loss
  - causes the development of eating disorders
  - triggers self-destructive thinking patterns, such as negative thoughts that lower self-esteem and a mentality that says, "I already blew it. Why not go all out and eat more?"
  - leads to self-defeating behaviors like prediet binges, stress eating, and automatic/unconscious eating
  - has effects that mimic the signs and symptoms of starvation

- Fat phobia and prejudice continue to fuel the diet industry. Despite its extremely low success rate among participants, it is a multibillion-dollar business.

- Drastic/rapid weight loss programs cause depletion of lean (desirable) muscle mass and a counterproductive metabolic reaction.

- The safest, most successful and permanent weight loss is gradual. Be patient with your body, and it will eventually learn to adjust to a healthier lifestyle for good.

~ 3 ~

Diets Gone Wild

According to the National Institute of Mental Health, one in five women struggles with either disordered eating behavior or an eating disorder.[1] Isn't that heart-wrenching? Whether you realize it or not, you're surrounded by eating-disordered individuals. They are your neighbors, your sister, yourself. Most of these people just suffer in silence as their diets fail and their metabolisms fizzle out. Only *one out of every ten* eating-disordered individuals receives treatment for the disorder.[2, 3]

It is true that far fewer men suffer from eating disorders. Estimates suggest that only 10 to 15 percent of the anorexic or bulimic population is male. However, when we contrast bulimic men with bulimic women, we find that the men tend to delay seeking treatment by an additional two years! It is also important to note that the proportion of males jumps up to 40 percent when we look at the binge-eating disorder population specifically.[4, 5] So even though men are less likely to fall into eating-disordered behavior, they are still susceptible, and the illness takes an equally detrimental toll on all affected individuals, no matter the gender.

As we discussed in the last chapter, people don't usually jump into an eating disorder with any malice in mind. Remember: eating disorders such as anorexia, bulimia, and binge-eating disorders are often the end result of—you guessed it—well-intended, seemingly harmless *dieting*, dieting that has gone terribly wrong.

At the beginning, dieters see their newfound self-discipline as something to be celebrated. They thrill over the satisfaction and fulfillment they get from their sacrificial endeavors. They jump for joy as the numbers on the scale drop, they feel elated as old clothes fit again and new clothes look great on their slimmer figures, and they savor the positive feedback that they receive from family and friends. Even better, the power of success elicits an "I hit the jackpot" kind of high.

The point is, nobody heads into a diet hoping to become anorexic. Eating disorders are essentially the best laid plans gone horribly awry. That's because once an eating disorder sets in, the dieters are no longer in charge. The disorder now controls *them*. Try as they might, eating disorder victims can't seem to separate themselves from their preoccupations with food or their cyclical patterns. They keep returning to dieting—the origin of the disorder—again and again, like a dog to his vomit. Over time, the initial success stories dissolve into pain, failure, and frustration.

Let's stop and take a look at the typical hallmark features of eating-disordered individuals. No matter what a person weighs or what form his or her disorder takes, every disordered-eating individual exhibits some commonalities.

You'll find the following:

- a diet plan that has gone terribly wrong
- a desire to be thin and attractive
- a feeling of powerlessness, a desire to get control of one's life
- an obsession with food
- sleep disturbances
- continued body dissatisfaction
- continued depression / augmentation of depressive symptoms
- continued fears of weight gain
- continued self-esteem issues

What do I mean by *continued* body dissatisfaction, depression, fears of weight gain, and self-esteem issues? Well, these issues aren't symptoms of the disorder; they were actually some of the causes. But they continue to persist despite the acquisition of a new weight or a thinner body.

The Development of the Eating Disorder

Ninety percent of eating-disordered individuals happen to be between the ages of twelve and twenty-five. That fact alone shows that something happens during adolescence that makes it the perfect breeding ground for developing an eating disorder. At age fourteen, only 28 percent of girls are engaged in some type of disordered-eating behavior. But by the time students reach college age, 60 percent have abnormal eating patterns.[7]

Why? What causes the sharp rise in disordered eating during adolescence? Here are some contributing factors:

- Adolescence is a time period filled with transitions and stressors. Depression and stress can both be causes for the development of eating disorders. Accordingly, the two peak periods of vulnerability for eating-disordered behavior are the transition into high school and the transition into college.[8]

- Parents fail to provide proper guidance regarding weight issues. They avoid addressing the issue of weight gain out of fear that their remarks will cause the future development of an eating disorder. Teenagers go with what they see in the tabloids, magazines, and TV ads; fad diets or dieting in general becomes the go-to solution. And as you now know, dieting initiates the onset of eating disorders.

- Teenagers are raised on a steady supply of carbohydrates. Delicious, addictive, concentrated sugar products with 24/7 availability create the perfect setup for addiction. Teens' palates become desensitized to the taste of sugar. Just like with any drug, larger doses are necessary for satiation. Excessive weight gain and consequent body dissatisfaction are the likely outcomes.

- Puberty hits at about the time girls reach one hundred pounds, which is happening at a younger and younger age (because of excessive carbohydrate intake).[9] At these young ages, girls are psychologically unprepared to be disciplined about their appearance. Before they know what's happened, girls can become heavy, pudgy, and unhappy with their bodies. Identity crises and low self-esteem emerge.

- Levels of estrogen and progesterone progressively increase as teens go through puberty. These hormones stimulate appetite and the development of secondary sex characteristics, which require the deposition of body fat. Most of the weight that is added during puberty goes on as body fat.

There is an epic eight-year study that is worth our while to examine here. Eric Stice, PhD, a senior research scientist at Oregon Research Institute, investigated predictors for the development of an eating disorder. Out of the four hundred middle school girls (with an average age of fourteen) that he followed, seventy-eight developed either a full-blown eating disorder or a subthreshold eating disorder. In other words, during those eight years, about one-fifth of the girls fell prey to the jaws of eating-disordered behavior!

Dr. Stice found three primary predictors for the development of an eating disorder,[10] presented here in order of importance:

1. body dissatisfaction
2. depressive symptoms
3. dieting behavior

Working backward, number 3 is further proof that dieting leads to disordered eating (as if we needed it!). As for number 2, we will return to the topic of depressive symptoms later on in the book. Let's take the time now to investigate number 1: body dissatisfaction, the leading predictor of eating disorder development.

Body Dissatisfaction

What is body dissatisfaction? Exactly who suffers from it?

According to the National Eating Disorders Association, 80 percent of American women are dissatisfied with their appearance.[11] Body dissatisfaction is almost universal.

A scene in the movie *Mean Girls* comically exemplifies the way many women think. Three of the main characters, all stunning young women, are standing in front of a mirror, tearing themselves apart. The newcomer to the group, Cady, grew up in Africa and isn't accustomed to the Western phenomenon of loathing one's own appearance.[12]

> Karen: My hips are huge!
> Gretchen: Oh please. I hate my calves.
> Regina: At least you guys can wear halters. I've got man shoulders.
> Cady (voiceover): I used to think there was just fat and skinny. But apparently there's lots of things that can be wrong on your body.
> Gretchen: My hairline is so weird.
> Regina: My pores are huge.
> Karen: My nail beds suck.
> (Pause. All look at Cady in expectation.)
> Cady (searching for something to add): I have really bad breath in the morning?
> Karen (looks disgusted): Ew!

We can laugh at this depiction, but the truth is it isn't too far from reality. Our society's obsession with beauty has led to unrealistic expectations for women and men alike. And these unrealistic expectations have, in turn, led to widespread body dissatisfaction.

From a young age, we learn to detest our features that fail to resemble the glorious gods and goddesses gracing our glamour magazines. Sixty-nine percent of girls in grades five through twelve state that images of models influence their idea of a perfect body shape.[13, 14] *Perfect?* Hmmm ... But the person staring back at us from the looking glass is perfectly *imperfect* in nearly every way. So when we compare that reflection to the chic, sexy, and fashionable stars on TV, how could we do anything but cringe at our reality?

Though body dissatisfaction is not gender specific, it hits the female sex particularly hard, especially at the beginning. Picture Barbie. That beautiful blond bombshell with huge eyes, perky breasts, a tiny waist, full lips, and long legs is the epitome of what we hope to be. As our five-year-old selves dressed our plastic childhood friends in sequins and heels, we never would have suspected the truth: this unrealistic, ideal female figurine was initiating us into a painful fantasy world.

This world only becomes more concrete as we mature and the beauty barrage intensifies. We are daily exposed to stick-thin women who magically have curves in all the right places. Whether consciously or unconsciously, we realize that this cosmetically altered figure is what we're supposed to strive for.

But real girls don't look like models. Nor will they ever be Barbie. You might have heard that if Barbie's exact proportions were recreated in a human being, she wouldn't even be able to stand up. A body like that is completely impractical; it's useless.

In order for a woman's body to function reproductively, it needs about 17 to 22 percent body fat. That's how we're meant to be. Men, on the other hand, only need 2 to 5 percent essentialto function![15] How unfair is that? Clearly, women were meant to have more fat on their bodies than men. Much of our extra fat lies just below the surface of our skin, in the subcutaneous layer. And while we may wish we could vacuum off this layer of fat, men like it. It makes us soft and lovable. But sadly, this silken layer of body fat also hides muscle tone. Thanks to estrogen and progesterone, we rarely ever see markedly defined muscles in women unless they're exercising or they are excessively thin.

Fashion models do have visible muscles, but it's not because they're athletes. Their toned look comes at a high price—starvation. The average model is 23 percent underweight, and many of them struggle with eating disorders.[16] Despite this fact, it is the model's slender and delicate figure that we aspire to achieve. Nowadays, even men are trained to value this fragile frame. Men want model-skinny girls with visible muscles and soft curves. But that combination doesn't even make sense physiologically.

Here's the nitty-gritty, everyday truth: the average female is five feet four inches tall and weighs 140 pounds, while the typical model is five feet eleven inches tall and weighs only 117 pounds! Fashion models are thinner than 98 percent of women.[17] That is plain unnatural!

In order to fight body dissatisfaction, we must—and I mean *must*— clean up our mistaken ideas about what constitutes the quintessential female. This ultra-thin, perfectly coiffured feminine archetype is terribly misleading for women. Our fantastical role models lead to feelings of inadequacy, a self-destructive inner voice, and much of our compensatory dieting behavior.

Let's be honest—most of us don't wake up looking runway ready. That's why cover girls and actresses undergo hours of beauty treatments. Even then, their images are photographed under controlled lighting and airbrushed so that they can remove any extra blemishes or cellulite. With an army of stylists, makeup artists, fashion consultants, and computer editors, our celebrities do look phenomenal. But in real life, these stars look rather normal.

The annoying part is that most preteen girls *do* sport the model-thin, svelte, athletic figure prior to the onslaught of hormones. They also have flawless skin, beautifully thick hair, and long, lean muscles. So the beauty queen standards might not seem too far out of reach at first. Then suddenly, out of the blue ... *Wham*! Puberty strikes, leaving behind unpredictable results. Breast buds, pimples, and hips ... er ... sprout? It takes years for the awkward phase to pass and the dust to settle.

The transition into a mature, womanly body necessitates huge *psychological* adjustments, as well. When we add to the biological, physical conundrum homework, sleep deprivation, driving accidents, missed curfews, control battles, family troubles, peer pressure, increasing levels of responsibility, and identity crises, despair and depression often follow.

In truth, body dissatisfaction is really a foil—an obsessive focus that distracts people from their true problems. Heck, it's not a bad idea when you think about it. Instead of stressing about real issues, like faulty self-esteem, depression, or family troubles, people ingeniously obsess over their large hips or big nose. Hours of one's life can be whittled away staring at imperfections. After all, it's easier to be a victim of life's cruel fate than to handle one's true failures.

So what can we do about it?

If you want to break free from frivolous obsessions over appearance and take on the challenge of real life, you will need to find a way to love the imperfect, authentic self. That means loving the person you see in the mirror—the one with acne, a flat chest, cankles, stringy hair ... whatever it is that you fixate your negative self-attention on. This is not a task for the faint of heart, and it is not accomplished overnight, but it can be done.

Now I have a very difficult question to ask: Is body dissatisfaction ever warranted, for example, with obesity?

Of course, our culture teaches ultimate tolerance, which is a very good thing most of the time. But I have to ask the rather taboo question: Shouldn't we realistically be dissatisfied with a doughy, out-of-shape body? *You bet.*

There *should* be dissatisfaction with anything (including weight) that leads to a myriad of long-term health problems. After all, discontentment is what instigates the desire for change, which leads to self-improving actions. Moreover, self-love and a rational dissatisfaction with weight *can* coexist. In fact, they actually belong together.

Loving the imperfect self does not mean that we should embrace being fat or obese. We should love ourselves enough to find healthier ways to live. After all, real self-love involves both nurturance and discipline.

Before we examine anorexia and bulimia nervosa in more detail, here is one more study concerning the predicting factors of eating disorders. Abbigail Tissot and her colleagues in the Division of Behavioral Medicine at Cincinnati Children's Hospital evaluated 871 girls, aged nine to ten, in hopes of determining what kinds of diets predispose children to eating disorders. Over a ten-year period, the subjects (and their parents) kept logs of their food intake. The study showed that the girls whose diets were *high in carbohydrates but low in fats* were at greatest risk for developing an eating disorder. By the age of fourteen, these girls were already suffering with more body dissatisfaction than the other girls.[18]

Tissot's study brings up a lot of tricky questions:

- Were the high-carb/low-fat eaters more insecure about their bodies because that kind of diet made them put on more weight?

- Do you think they were more likely to develop an eating disorder because a high-carb/low-fat diet leads to body fat deposition in the least desirable areas?

- Could their body dissatisfaction be connected to the blood sugar swings of a high-carb diet?

- Were they more dissatisfied with themselves because their diets lacked fats, which are natural mood-stabilizers?

- Are girls who limit fats the ones who are already more obsessed with weight and diet and the ones who are already predisposed to have an eating disorder?

Wow. That's a lot of food for thought. Maybe these are all factors that need to be considered. We'll address these issues in more detail when we examine how our bodies use various food groups. But in the meantime, it wouldn't hurt to ponder the connection between low-fat/high-carb diets and body dissatisfaction.

Anorexia Nervosa

"5–10% of anorexics die within ten years of onset, 18–20% die within twenty years of onset, and only 50% report ever being cured."[19]

"20% of people suffering from anorexia will prematurely die from complications related to their eating disorder, including suicide and heart problems."[20]

Anorexia nervosa is the deadliest mental illness out there. It has the highest death rate because of the myriad of medical complications, associated medical disorders, and completed suicides.

The hallmark signs and symptoms of anorexia nervosa are the following:

- low body weight: less than 85 percent of normal weight for height and age
- intense fear of weight gain
- restriction of calories and fats, reduction of food intake
- denial of hunger, denial of illness
- distorted view of one's body weight[21, 22]
- abnormal patterns of handling food
- purging behavior through the use of exercise, laxatives, or diuretics. (This may or may not be present.)

- amenorrhea in women (They don't get their period—hormones and reproductive functioning are altered and stopped in the face of starvation. Remember, women need to have 18 to 22 percent body fat in order to menstruate.)

Think way, way back … all the way to the last chapter when we discussed the signs and symptoms of semistarvation. Do you recognize how similar the symptoms of anorexia are to those of semistarvation? It makes sense. Anorexia nervosa is the result of self-imposed starvation.

This disorder requires ultimate control: a totalitarian dictatorship of both mind and body. One needs to resist every instinctual impulse to eat—impulses that never stop and even get louder over time. But once the tyrant inside has initiated its reign of terror, the anorexic can go on autopilot. The disease develops a life of its own.

As the restriction of food progresses, the anorexic's body begins to compensate for the lack of available nutrition. It shuts down. Any unnecessary body functions (like menstruation) are terminated. The metabolic rate drops. The circulating level of thyroid hormone decreases. Blood pressure drops. The pulse slows. Skin becomes dry and flaky. Nails become brittle. Constipation becomes a frequent problem. And the list goes on. Again, this is an innate survival mechanism. God made the body selectively protect two things, the brain and the heart, for as long as it possibly can. Everything else takes the backseat.

Without any fat to keep them warm, anorexics develop a fine, downy-like layer of *lanugo* hair. But even this extra lanugo hair cannot prevent the cold sensitivity or the drop in body temperature that is seen in anorexics. They simply have nothing to burn for thermal energy. Eventually, fuel for living comes from organ tissue: the liver, kidneys, heart, and brain. In other words, the body starts eating itself since it has nothing else to eat. Finally, the heart muscle becomes weak and damaged. Death most commonly results from muscular failure or electrical problems of the heart. Anorexics literally die of a broken heart.

Neuroimaging studies have provided evidence of the changes that take place in the anorexic's starved brain. What is seen is a global reduction of gray matter and enlargement of cerebrospinal fluid spaces and cortical sulci, all of which point to a loss of brain tissue. This means that you can't and won't think well. The pituitary gland (an important regulator of hormonal function) shrinks too. Some of these changes may be permanent.[23]

If you're thinking, *Why would anyone inflect such drastic damage on him- or herself? And who would want to look that skinny, anyway? A hollowed-out, eighty-five pound skeleton is not my idea of beautiful*, then count yourself fortunate, because your reasoning is still intact. Once a body becomes emaciated, reasoning goes out the window. It's as if a virus takes over the software of the anorexic's brain, making it impossible for her to free herself from bizarre behaviors and thoughts. When the anorexic looks in the mirror and stares at the skeleton she has become, she still obsesses over the tiny bit of fat that is evident only to her. Until there is a refeeding process, therapy is fairly futile.

People assume that anorexics get so good at refusing food that it gets easier and easier. Maybe they stop feeling hungry altogether at some point. *Nope.* And I'll show you why.

Many neurohormones and neuropeptides are altered in eating-disordered patients, most likely as a consequence of their peculiar eating habits. Two key hormones play a role in maintaining the anorexic's large appetite. Neuropeptide Y is elevated in anorexics. This chemical makes a well-fed laboratory rat continue eating to the point of being stuffed, far in excess of its needs. Don't believe the anorexic who tells you she is not hungry. Anorexics' hunger can be overwhelming, which freaks them out to no end. They fear that if they start eating, they won't be able to stop. So their excessive hunger propels them into even tighter control.

Leptin is another hormone that is messed up in anorexics. It comes from fat cells. Since they don't have any fat, their leptin levels are very low. This is really unfortunate, because leptin suppresses appetite. So when leptin levels are low, as they are in anorexics and bulimics, hunger is not suppressed, which leads to an increased appetite and, in most people, an increase in food intake. Low leptin levels may also inhibit reproductive function. Sometimes menses (a girl's period) never returns.

Another key hormone that misbehaves in anorexics is cortisol—the stress hormone. Cortisol levels are elevated in people suffering from anorexia, depression, or chronic stress disorders. Elevated cortisol levels lead to muscle wasting, central fat deposition (!!), hyposexuality, and hyperactivity. *Hyper*activity. You'd think they'd be slow and sluggish without fuel, but they actually have an awful nervous energy that makes them restless, agitated, and fidgety.

I don't want to overwhelm you, but please hang in there as I cover two last, very important hormones that are off-kilter in anorexics: vasopressin and oxytocin. (Last two! Almost there!)

Vasopressin is a cool hormone because it enhances memory function. Wow, give me some of that stuff, right? Well, in anorexics we find that this hormone *is* elevated. But guess what; in anorexics, this is not a good thing. It contributes to their uncanny ability to train themselves to respond to negative conditioning. It perpetuates their odd obedience to their crazy, invented rules, like "If I even think about eating cake, I'm gonna make myself brush my teeth," or "Since I ate that piece of pizza, I need to run around the house ten times and do one hundred sit-ups. Now I'll learn never to make that mistake again." And that really happens.

Meanwhile, oxytocin (nicknamed the cuddle hormone) is decreased. Oxytocin is a hormone that leads to bonding and relaxation. It's elevated in women after they deliver a baby; it lets them chill out and not be neurotic about details. Because its level is so low in anorexics, their already uptight, guarded, obsessive, and rigid behaviors intensify. No cuddling for them. Definitely not cuddle bunnies.

Do you see how we have a neurochemical soup that is the perfect recipe for disaster? With oxytocin at low levels and vasopressin at high levels, anorexics are naturally capable of maintaining their obsessive rituals. They can out-willpower anyone. They defy reason and rescue.

You can see why refeeding is essential for treatment, and why this serious disorder needs medical attention as soon as it is recognized. Even with treatment, the anorexic's prognosis is not good. Many of them repeatedly relapse back into their disorder throughout their lives. They become masters of self-denial and sacrifice until finally they succumb to their obsession's final demand—death.[24, 25, 26]

Bulimia Nervosa

Bulimia is a disorder that is associated with persistent dieting and an excessively negative body image. Bulimics, like anorexics, have a fear of weight gain that leads them to restrict calories. But unlike anorexics, bulimics find themselves giving in to their hunger cravings. They engage in numerous episodes of unrestrained bingeing—bingeing that's followed by physical pain, disgust, and self-loathing. They cannot take the weighty consequences of their gluttony. Purging, through exercise, vomiting, laxatives, or diuretics becomes a necessity. Before long, the bulimic finds him- or herself slipping into repeated cycles of starvation, bingeing, guilt, and purging.

Have you ever seen anyone bingeing on radishes and artichokes? Probably not. Bulimics usually indulge in foods that are rich in carbohydrates and fat. During a binge, the bulimic escapes into a numbed, dissociative state. Stress and awareness of the here and now become blunted. It's a bit like the famous story of Dr. Jekyll and Mr. Hyde. Dr. Jekyll would wake up not remembering where he had been the night before. But the evidence of his crimes gave clues to his mysterious behavior. Dr. Jekyll's dark side, Mr. Hyde, took over at night and did things he would never have done in his right mind. Well, that's a really exaggerated metaphor for what happens to bulimics. Before they know it, they're staring at an empty ice cream carton, a hollow cookie jar, and bare cupboards. Bulimics can easily consume days' worth of leftovers or an entire cake within a half hour. After depleting the kitchen of choice foods, they might mindlessly move on to less desirable food—sometimes even resorting to gross things like Crisco oil or dry, uncooked spaghetti noodles! Imagine Dr. Jekyll's guilt after a bingeing episode like that.

Bulimics obsess about food. They count and restrict calories, put themselves through grueling exercise routines, plan meals, and even plan binges. For example, an ice skater might think, *I'll starve myself until the competition so I look good in my costume. And then afterward, I'll bake a cake and eat the entire thing by myself as a reward.*

The vast majority of binges occur privately, when the bulimic is alone or while everyone else is asleep. Bulimics don't want their feasts to be soured by others' judgment. They can't risk discovery. But despite all their attempts at secrecy, discovery does occur. The after-meal trips to the bathroom are definitely more than coincidental. The sound of retching gives them away. The absence of an entire cheesecake from the refrigerator is too strange. And the obligatory, strenuous, punitive, daily workouts are surefire signs.

Contributing Factors for Bulimia

Who is vulnerable to developing bulimia or binge-eating disorder? Or put differently, why do these illnesses occur?

D-I-E-T-S. Dieting is the perfect setup for the development of eating-disordered behavior. In 1981, researchers found that dieting preceded the onset of bulimia in 88 percent of their study's sample group.[27] In 1967, another researcher found that the longer patients have been starved, the more likely they are to experience binges.[28] And in 1978, another study showed that the breakdown of control occurs about nine months after the onset of dieting.[29] So people are able to restrict and regulate their diets for about as long as it takes to have a baby. By the time the bun is fully cooked, dieters burn out; binges begin.

Granted, there are other factors that contribute to vulnerability to these disorders, such as psychological issues, genetics, depression, anxiety, and social stressors. But dieting itself is usually the match that starts the fire.

By this point, we pretty much have our recipe for bulimia. Ingredients: a pinch of stress, a touch of self-abuse, a dash of anger, a helping of bad genetics, a splash of insecurity, a hefty dose of impulsivity, a measure of starvation, and a cup of depression. Sift these dry ingredients together. Pour the mixture into an empty bowl of DIET. Wet it all down with a little corn syrup and voila! *Bulimia a la ad nauseam.* A peculiarly disastrous culinary dish.

Just like any other recipe, once a person has learned it, very little thought is necessary for its recreation. The recipe for disaster becomes a go-to plan whenever escape or penance is necessary.

Despite, or even because of, all the self-abusive purging techniques that bulimics employ, they often struggle with maintaining a thin, healthy weight.

Why? Why aren't bulimics stick thin?

It all has to do with the physiology of the GI tract and the way our bodies absorb the food we eat. Let me explain why bulimics are shooting themselves in the foot with their weight-regulation tactics.

First off, carbohydrate digestion begins in the mouth. So sugar is the first thing to be assimilated into the body. Fats, proteins, and fiber-rich food take much longer to be digested, absorbed, and utilized. So when people chew on food for the taste and then spit it out quickly, they are still absorbing some of the sugar and other simple carbohydrates! Same goes for purgers. They absorb the simple carbohydrates through their mouths and stomachs and vomit up the protein, fat, and fiber. In short, their plan backfires; they take in the worst parts of food and reject all the good ingredients.

The simple carbohydrates that are absorbed immediately trigger an insulin response that is appropriate for the load ingested, even though most of it is about to be purged. That large amount of insulin tucks the sugars away into storage (a.k.a. fat). Then, when the protein, fat, fiber, minerals, and vitamins are vomited up, hunger returns. It's the worst of both worlds. The bulimic takes in the sugar, turns it into fat, *and* is left with an empty tummy, hungry for more.

Laxatives are also dangerously appealing. They're relatively cheap, the results are quick, and the temporary rewards of perceived weight loss can be measured on scales. However, these pills are masters of deception. In the long-term, the result of laxative use isn't a flat stomach but rather, a very messed-up, flabby colon.

The colon's job is very different from that of the stomach and the small intestine. It absorbs vitamins and liquid and concentrates feces. Laxatives work by poisoning the muscles of the colon, causing massive spasms and a fast transit of material out of the large intestine. Remember, by the time food reaches the intestines, all of the carbohydrate calories have been absorbed. So very few calories, if any, are lost by using laxatives. Then what is lost? Water, fiber, and electrolytes—*not* calories.

Have you ever had messed-up electrolytes because of profuse sweating or vomiting? If so, you know how weak and confused you can feel. Anytime that we are two to five pounds off in our fluid balance, we feel pretty disgusting. This isn't weight loss; it's self-inflicted misery!

Thanks to a study done in 1983, we have an actual measurement of the ineffectiveness of laxatives. Bo-Lynn and colleagues had their subjects consume nearly two thousand calories before taking fifty Correctol tablets. That's a lot of calories and *a lot* of tablets. The desired effect of diarrhea was achieved from the laxative ingestion. Over 6.3 quarts of liquid were lost on average! But following the diarrhea, only 12 percent of the calories were removed, about two hundred calories in all.[30] After taking *fifty* tablets? That's it?

Laxative users buy into this fake weight loss. They rejoice at the falling numbers on the scale. In order to maintain it, they restrict fluid and salt. You see, salt can cause water retention, especially in people who are protein deficient or are abusing diuretics or laxatives. The body naturally wants to hold on to any fluid and electrolytes it gets in order to replenish what was lost. Furthermore, it naturally tries to prepare for the next bout of drug-abuse that will cause even more fluid loss. So the bodies of laxative abusers retain water and the scale numbers go right back up.

Over time, laxative abusers need higher and higher doses of pills to achieve the same result. They become hooked on the drug—addicted. Not only do they need the laxatives to prevent their weight from increasing, but worse yet, they actually need the laxatives to defecate. That's because their bowels become weak, flabby, enlarged, and unresponsive. The intestines and colon can't do their jobs on their own anymore. Constipation becomes a huge problem, necessitating weekly enemas just to poop. Long-term abusers need to get on a supervised bowel regimen. That's how much they have messed up their bodies. I once had a female patient who could only have a bowel movement if and when she took her thirty-six Ex-Lax tablets. She regularly scheduled a day off from work so that she could be near a bathroom. Shockingly, she was actually a nurse and thus knew all about the dangers of laxative misuse!

When laxative abusers attempt to get off their drug, they often complain of edema or significant fluid retention. For weeks, even months after the discontinuation of laxatives, the abuser has to deal with a full gut and constipation, *plus* pounds of puffiness. It's a miserable and discouraging recovery period, so they often return to their pathologic addiction.

We should never let the scale be our guide to physical health. It naturally fluctuates by up to five pounds per day, depending on hormones, the time of day, bowel movements, and salt intake. But the fluctuations experienced by laxative abusers are huge; the ups and downs of the scale are much more extreme. That's just another contributing factor to their tendency to relapse.

Bulimia sounds like a terrible disorder, doesn't it? I'm sure you're smart enough to want to steer clear of it now. But what if you suspect that a friend is suffering from this disorder? How would you know?

Let's look at the physical repercussions of bulimia that may help alert you to a friend in need. Constant vomiting causes swollen salivary glands in the cheeks along with mouth and throat sores. You might see scars, calluses, sores, and swelling on hands and knuckles. (Stomach acid not only erodes their insides, but it also erodes the hands that force them to gag.) Because stomach acid destroys enamel, teeth might lose their whiteness. You could even see tooth decay and the loss of teeth. Fatigue and dry skin are also typical symptoms.

If you're worried that a friend has a problem, let your genuine love and concern be your guide. If the problem appears serious, let your friend know that you need to help him or her and reach out to a family member, a therapist, or a trusted colleague. Then please follow through. I know it's hard, but it's better to have an angry friend who's alive than a best buddy who succumbs to his or her illness.

Before we finish this discussion, I'd like to highlight the most serious and disturbing side effects and complications associated with bulimia nervosa, not to upset you, but to show you why this illness is far more dangerous than many people realize.

- gastrointestinal disturbances—Recurrent vomiting leads to a weakened esophageal sphincter, thus allowing food to pass easily between the stomach and the esophagus. It becomes so easy, in fact, that food will start to come up with just a burp or a cough! This horribly easy regurgitation of food may help perpetuate the disorder and lead to further irritation of the already irritated and inflamed esophagus. Rupture of the stomach or esophagus can lead to death. More frequent are stomach enlargement, esophagitis, and esophageal tears.

- neurological problems—These include seizures, muscle spasms, and tingling and numbness of the extremities.

- kidney dysfunction—Kidney problems are most likely due to chronically low potassium levels and dehydration from purging.

- menstrual irregularities—Menstrual irregularities are reported in anywhere from 50 to 90 percent of bulimics. Because of alternating starvation and binges, even normal-weight bulimics can stop getting their period.

- edema and dehydration—Dieting, vomiting, and diuretic or laxative abuse lead to periods of dehydration and then a rebound of water retention. Low blood pressure, feelings of dizziness, tremendous thirst, and decreased urinary output are likely to follow. As I mentioned previously, the body holds on to fluid, resulting in puffiness in the fingers, ankles, and face.

- enlarged paralytic colon and constipation—Laxatives, such as phenothaline products or senna products, contain compounds that damage the nerve cells responsible for muscle contraction in the colon. Over time, more and more laxatives are necessary for bowel movements. The end result is a flabby colon and constipation.

- emotional issues—A general lack of psychological well-being is described and includes feelings of shame and inadequacy, anxiety, depression, sleep disturbance, and general malaise.

- arrhythmias and sudden death—Electrolyte imbalances may cause weakness and muscle cramping all over the body. Remember, the heart is a muscle, so it becomes very prone to arrhythmias (irregular nerve and muscle firing) whenever the balance of fluid and electrolytes is disturbed. Ipecac, often used to induce vomiting, can also cause muscle weakness and cardiac abnormalities, adding to the risk for heart failure. Imagine a weak and dysfunctional heart trying to function while pushed through a bulimic's strenuous exercise routine. Stressing the heart through exercise can lead to significant cardiac abnormalities.[32, 33, 34, 35]

Have you heard enough? This is *scary* stuff, to say the least, nothing to mess around with! People with any eating disorder often spend years in and out of hospitals and a lifetime trying to recover.

You have now read the psychiatric criteria for bulimia nervosa and anorexia nervosa. But as you've probably figured out, many people don't fit into one of these strict categories. It's not all black and white; there are loads of gray areas. Many anorexics have bulimic symptoms, and a large number of obese people binge. Furthermore, loads of individuals simply live with disordered eating on a daily basis. Some people chew food and spit it out. Some people slip in and out of bulimia and anorexia. Some people simply binge eat and don't purge.

How about diet pills? Many people who might not otherwise be considered bulimic or anorexic use them, and they are probably even more mainstream than laxatives. How do these drugs affect the body?

Diet pills come in many forms. Many are uppers, giving the user a sudden burst of energy and loss of appetite. But what happens when the drug is out of your system? You can always expect the exact opposite behavior to occur—in this case, sluggishness and hunger. So people take more. Eventually, they become tolerant to the uppers and need more and more to feel energetic and to quell their hunger. Hmmm ... all of this makes diet pills sound eerily similar to cocaine.

As if this weren't enough, diet pills cause the depletion of neuro-chemicals. They can be highly addictive and can lead to further problems with arrhythmias and increase the risk for sudden death.

The point is pathologic eating of any kind, including the use of diet pills, is detrimental. That's why the categories and criteria for anorexia and bulimia are not the determinants for who needs help. Every person out there who struggles with pathologic patterns of eating deserves to learn how to manage their health. Every person who exhibits disordered eating deserves the supervision and medical care that leads to wellness.

I have to be honest though; even with professional help, only about half of patients completely recover.[36] Why? Because recovery from any eating disorder is very difficult, both physically and psychologically.

Recall, if you will, the men in Ancel Keyes's study, whom we considered in the previous chapter (the thirty-six men who volunteered as an alternative to military service in 1950). When they were allowed to return to normal eating, they overshot the threshold for what is considered healthy by about 10 percent. That's the norm for recovering individuals. You see, excessive weight gain is a natural follow-up to dieting and starvation because the body doesn't trust its owner; it has become paranoid that he or she will inflict another round of diet pills, laxatives, or starvation at any moment. Unsurprisingly, it's on the defensive after such maltreatment.

Imagine how upsetting it would be, as a weight-obsessed person, to weigh even more after treatment than you did when you started dieting. The hospital staff may be rejoicing over their patient's healthy weight, but secretly, the chronic dieter can't wait to leave treatment and return to his or her dieting behavior. Relapses become all too common, which only further disrupts the body and delays recovery even more.

Patience. That's what the road to recovery requires. And a large dose of character strength wouldn't go amiss either. With time, the body's neurochemicals rebalance and its metabolism improves, but there's no way to get around this difficult transition period. It takes about a year of healthy eating for the body to regain trust in its owner and allow its weight to return to its normal *set point.*

Set Point
*the weight around which your body naturally hovers

Is there such a thing as a set point? Our genes determine our bone structure and body shape, but are they *the* determining factor in weight maintenance as well? In other words, are we destined to have the same body figure as our parents and ancestors?

It does seem that our bodies want to rest at their own predetermined weights, as if they were protecting a particular body habitus, whether heavy or thin. This may be why it's so difficult for people to change their weight and body figure, no matter what they do. However, it's also true that we pick up eating habits and preferences from our parents, and these do *not* have to be our destiny. We may not be able to alter our genetics, but we *can* alter our eating choices. How much of a difference can healthy choices make in our set point?

Fortunately, a great deal. Studies have shown that although genetics determines our general body habitus, diet and lifestyle choices can alter our set point within certain limits.

To lower your set point:

1. Regularly participate in aerobic exercise. Move your body; don't be a couch potato.[37]
2. Avoid sugar/fat combination foods: mixed coffee drinks, milkshakes, smoothies, candy bars, ice cream, doughnuts, cake, cookies, muffins, cinnamon rolls, etc.
3. Also minimize plain sugar sources: candy, sugar drinks, sorbet, jelly, Jell-O, pudding ...[38]
4. Choose only high-fiber, low-glycemic-index carbohydrates (more on this in chapter 4).
5. Take in adequate amounts of protein and healthy fat each day.
6. Get enough sleep, roughly eight hours.[39]
7. Reduce stress levels.[40]
8. Whatever you do, don't diet. Yo-yo (on and off) dieting raises your set point.

Finding the healthy, lean weight that is right for your body is important. But you never want to focus so much on lowering your set point that you are teetering on the edge of health. Don't test the lower limits. It's way too risky, too easy to drop off the edge into an eating disorder.

The Athlete's Challenge

Many athletes, including wrestlers, runners, divers, skiers, horse jockeys, rowers, and most notably dancers, gymnasts, and figure skaters, have no choice but to walk this tightrope, always vulnerable to falling into anorexia. The professional, aesthetic, and technical demands of their crafts leave them little choice. That's why, compared with the national eating disorders rate of about 3 percent,[41] elite athletes present with a rate as high as 13.5 percent.[42] Breaking this stat down even further, we learn that the prevalence among male collegiate athletes is around 20 percent and among female collegiate athletes, 25 percent.[43] According to the Eating Disorders Hope organization, "42 percent of female athletes competing in *aesthetic* sports demonstrated eating disordered behaviors."[44] Perhaps worst of all, one study even found that 83 percent of ballet dancers meet the criteria for chronic or lifetime eating disorders.[45]

Since these Herculean individuals are suffering at an extraordinarily high rate, I think it vital to specifically address the unique challenges of avoiding an eating disorder as an elite athlete. I'll also briefly zero in on the dance industry because that's where we observe the highest rates of all.

*Disclaimer: The following information is based on generalizations; of course, there is a great deal of variation within the elite athlete population. However, these generalizations come from countless athletes' words and experiences along with studies that focus on the particularities of this demographic.

Elite athletes like their bodies to feel like a finely tuned machine over which they have total control. Ideally, they prefer to maintain just enough muscle to perform optimally and nothing more, so that they aren't weighed down by extra baggage. Accordingly, a fear of body fat can develop not just for aesthetic reasons, but also because of the physics of what they do.

What kind of personality does the crème de la crème of physical activity usually possess? Let's see ... astounding self-control, an incredibly high pain tolerance, a competitive streak, a tendency toward self-criticism, obsessive-compulsive behavioral traits, perfectionism, the ability to sacrifice immediate gratification for long-term rewards ... In short, everything you need to excel in most endeavors, including destructive ones like restrictive eating. For the immensely disciplined athlete, ignoring hunger or engaging in obsessive eating rituals is no different than pushing through the tenth kilometer of the race. The show must go on; who cares if your toenail just fell off? No pain no gain, or as others say, "Pain is weakness leaving the body." This is the mentality that perpetuates masochistic tendencies—in dieting as well as exercising.

To add fuel to the fire, top athletes face innumerable external pressures. Weigh-ins for rowers and wrestlers, for instance, can cause dangerous and extreme behaviors. The practice of "cutting weight" just before a weigh-in often involves the combination of drastic dehydration, fasting, and grueling workouts. In 1998, three collegiate wrestlers died from extreme weight-control behavior, which led the National Collegiate Athletic Association (NCAA) to add six pounds to each weight class, enforce a minimum weight based on body fat composition, and change weigh-in procedures for competitions.[46]

Across the board, coaches, teachers, and employers often implicitly and explicitly pressure athletes to maintain an extremely low weight. This is true despite the fact that malnourishment increases both the frequency of injuries and the recovery time.[47] That means that in many ways, authority figures and athletes are shooting themselves in the foot by perpetuating the culture of undernourishment, because in the long run, ill health significantly impedes performance quality and the ability to perform at all.

I must be careful to point out that we can't place all of the blame on coaches and employers, especially when it comes to aesthetic sports (or athletic arts), such as figure skating and dance. Those in charge are obeying even higher masters: their audience and their customer base. Whether consciously or unconsciously, audience members prefer the aesthetic of waif-thin dancers and figure skaters who seem like they float and whose limbs go on forever. The loudest voices belong to the critics. Take for example the *New York Times* dance critic who wrote in a review of a New York City ballet dancer, she "looked as if she'd eaten one sugar plum too many."[48] Appropriately, this vicious comment produced a very public uproar, but similarly hurtful statements go unnoticed all the time.

If these are the opinions that employers, coaches, and teachers must cater to, it's hardly surprising that they promote the athletes/ performers who fit their spectators' preferred mold. Researchers E. L. Lowenkopf and L. M. Vincent found evidence of this in the ballet industry and published the following statement in the *Hillside Journal of Clinical Psychiatry*: "Professional dancers linked their physical appearance with a system of rewards and sanctions in which weight-gain led to non-selection for parts and negative reinforcement, whilst weight-loss was linked with praise and selection."[49, 50] In other words, the dancers in their studies knew that they had to lose weight or stay extremely thin in order to further their career. You might wonder how the people in charge get away with this harmful behavior. Well, the system of rewards and sanctions for weight control is conveniently implicit; the puppet-masters can justify casting or employment decisions with a million reasons and vehemently deny that weight has anything to do with it. Consequently, it's surprisingly easy for them to publicly condemn unhealthy eating patterns with their words while reinforcing them with their actions behind the scenes.

Both men and women in these career paths face the challenges of stringent weight control, yet women undeniably have it harder. The facts of biology mean that they mature at a younger age than their male counterparts, yet the facts of their career paths mean that they have to stay skinnier than the boys and men who lift them above their heads. What an impossible dilemma for a young, aspiring ballerina to deal with! If they choose health, they may have to deal with the humiliation of not being able to participate in partnered dance or the shame of dancing with boys who grunt and shake in the effort to lift them. The *easier* decision in this perverse situation might be to stave off puberty for as long as possible. True, this means giving up normal body functioning, but at least the individual gets to dance. When that's all you care about in life, you're willing to pay any price.

The result is that 40 percent of ballet dancers meet the criteria for anorexia nervosa at any given time, and the rate of amenorrhea and irregular menses is as high as 47 percent.[51] Lowenkopf and Vincent go as far as characterizing the dance industry as "the most obsessively weight-conscious subculture in [the] country."[52]

Surely there must be people in this competitive field who can keep their heads above the fray and maintain a healthy body image and weight, right? Of course! It's as simple as pie, actually. All you have to do as a dancer is this: never look at yourself in the mirrors that line the walls of your workplace; never compare yourself to your colleagues, who are also wearing skin-tight or minimal clothing; give no heed to the costume designers who take your measurements, reading out numbers and writing them down next to your coworkers'; ignore the commonplace physical exams of health-care professionals who check your weight and body fat percentage; ignore the almost constant flow of comments like, "I feel fat today," or "This mirror/costume makes me look huge"; and train yourself not to care at all about casting or job promotions. Easy, right?

Maybe for a handful of people blessed with iron strong self-confidence it's easy, but I personally won't blame the dancers who find it nearly impossible to see these high-pressured circumstances as no big deal when it's their reality, day after day.

The bottom line is this: elite athletes, no matter what field they're in, aren't given the luxury of maintaining a comfortable buffer zone between thinness and anorexia. They have to walk the tightrope, *but*— and this is a huge *but*—there is no good excuse for having an eating disorder, because there is no good excuse for demolishing one's mental and physical health.

Top athletes may be exceptional in many ways, but they are *not* exceptional biologically. Eating disorders destroy them from the inside out, just like they would anyone else. When anorexia is closing in on a victim, it will not stop and say, "Oh, you're an athlete? My bad! I won't bother you since I know you're facing different pressures to stay skinny than most people, and that's just not fair. So here's a free pass; I'll ignore all the physical signs that tell me your body is famished and in a state of emergency. I'll let you sneak by without slowly killing you."

No. We are all equal before the eyes of anorexia.

So if you're an elite athlete, what are you to do?

Prioritize long-term health over career advancement, no matter what. Admittedly, this may involve making difficult choices, perhaps passing up opportunities. But *nothing* is worth more than the one body you have, the one that must last you for decades after your career ends. That is priceless.

If you are to withstand destructive pressures within your industry, you'll need support. It helps to have support from friends, family members, and coworkers, but the most important person to have on your side is yourself. If ever you have to go through the disappointment (God forbid) of watching peers pass you by because they are willing to jeopardize their bodies in order to fit an inhuman aesthetic ideal, you need to be your number-one fan for not following their lead. Congratulate yourself on winning the best prize of all, lifelong health. Don't rely on external recognition; supply your own positive reinforcement.

You can also take heart in knowing that you are championing the cause of health in your sport for future athletes, as well as yourself. After all, changing a culture of destructive eating patterns can only come from within any given field. I, as a psychiatrist and eating disorders specialist, cannot transform your industry. But you can. You can be the living proof that you do *not* need to choose between health and athletic excellence. You *can* have both.

There will be tangible benefits to your wisdom, too. For one thing, your energy, stamina, and strength will be vastly improved with proper nutrition, and as I briefly mentioned before, your likelihood of injury will decrease, as will the length of time it takes for you to recover.[53] So in the long run, you'll essentially be a walking embodiment of the Daft Punk song lyrics: "harder, better, faster, stronger."

****

What should you take away from a chapter full of frightening statistics and dire warnings?

If nothing else, I hope you conclude that dieting is dangerous and that no matter who you are—athlete, figure skater, overworked mom or dad, high-strung college student, you name it—you endeavor to steer clear of anything that even resembles disordered eating for the rest of your life. Thankfully, steady, healthy eating alone will gradually and safely bring you to a lean weight.

Summary
Diets Gone Wild

- One in five women struggles with an eating disorder, yet only one in ten ever receive treatment.

- Although men make up only 10 percent of the total eating disorders population, when it comes to binge-eating disorder, they suffer at nearly the same rate as women.

- No one chooses to develop an eating disorder. Psychologically stable and unstable people are equally vulnerable to this group of diseases.

- The top three precipitating factors for the development of an eating disorder are depression, body dissatisfaction, and dieting. These and other issues (like feelings of powerlessness and self-esteem problems) continue or increase in severity through the duration of the eating disorder.

- Adolescence is a particularly vulnerable period of life for the development of an eating disorder.

- Only about half of eating disorder victims ever achieve full recovery.

- Eating disorders can be deadly. Within twenty years of the onset of anorexia, 10 to 20 percent of its victims die.

- The neurochemical changes that take place in the body as a result of an eating disorder often perpetuate the disease.

- Eating disorder victims develop obsessions and compulsive rituals and experience sleep disruption, agitation, hyposexuality, and hyperactivity because of semistarvation and the related nutritional deficiencies.

- Bulimic behaviors are counterproductive.

- Purging and excessive exercise increase appetite.

- Vomiting eliminates only the nutritive elements of food, rather than those that deposit fat because the body absorbs simple sugars very quickly.

- The medical complications of purging behaviors are serious and deadly.

- Eating disorders, like snakes, swallow their victims whole. Early and proactive intervention is crucial in order to save vulnerable and affected individuals.

- Athletes are much more susceptible than the general population to falling prey to eating disorders. About 13.5 percent of elite athletes suffer from an eating disorder, and the highest reported proportion is among ballet dancers, with as much as 83 percent meeting lifetime criteria for the set of illnesses.

- Employers, authority figures, coaches, fans, audience members, and critics all explicitly and implicitly pressure athletes to maintain extremely low weights despite the fact that malnourishment increases the frequency of injuries and recovery time.

- We need more athletes championing the cause of health. Prioritizing long-term health over career advancement is essential.

- No one should suffer long-term damage for the sake of his or her sport or career.

~ 4 ~

How Our Bodies Use Food

A calorie is the approximate amount of energy required to raise the temperature of one kilogram of water by one degree Celsius.

Sounds pretty exact. So when we measure our food in calories, it doesn't matter whether we get 100 calories from cake or from walnuts; a calorie is a calorie is a calorie. Right? *Wrong.*

Measuring food by calories is incredibly misleading because the body absolutely *does not* treat 100 calories of spinach the same as 100 calories of cake. That's why diets that rely on a calorie limit, say 1,500 per day, are pretty much useless. And those 100-calorie snack packs? That's good that you're eating *less* junk food. But your body isn't fooled; you're still eating junk food, and it will treat it as such.

When I ran an eating disorders clinic, I had many patients who illustrated this point perfectly. However, three women in particular created lasting impressions on me. Though I have changed their names here, their stories are entirely authentic.

Diana was a normal-weight seventeen-year-old who went on a 400-calorie white rice diet. Rose, an overweight twenty-year-old, ate only about 600 calories of fruit every day. Though the third woman, a very large-boned, middle-aged schoolteacher named Leslie, allowed herself a bit more variety, she still stuck to simple carbohydrates in her measly 400-calorie diet.

Why did these three women choose simple carbohydrates? First, because they liked the taste. Simple carbs are yummy, and they're comfort food, so people often choose to give up everything else rather than their simple carbs, even when they hear this is the very food group that leads to weight gain. And secondly, they knew that carbohydrates are only 4 calories per gram. Protein is as well, but they'd been taught to fear animal fats, and fats are 9 calories per gram, so heaven forbid they ingest any of *those*. These women had been fooled by the "fat on the lips equals fat on the hips" mythology.

At 400 to 600 calories per day, Diana, Rose and Leslie were inflicting misery upon themselves, and yet they still didn't lose weight. Do you find this hard to believe? I certainly did … I thought they must be leaving out secret binges from their food journals. But when I saw that their vital signs were terribly messed up, I realized that they were probably giving me an accurate account. They all had a slow pulse, such low blood pressure that they felt faint when they stood up, and lab results reflective of their low protein intake (with signs of a weakened immune system and heart and respiratory system dysfunction). Worse yet, they all seemed depressed, emotionally flat, colorless in complexion, and mentally dulled.

Though their diets were absolutely failing them, it was still very difficult to convince these women that they would actually burn more calories and feel 100 percent better if they balanced their energy intake. In other words, they needed to stop fearing protein and fat and they needed to eat more calories.

Did you know that the act of eating raises metabolism? Well, neither did Diana, Rose, or Leslie. But it's true; eating burns calories. Breaking down food and sorting through its components requires energy. So eating more often leads to a faster and more efficient metabolism. Eating less often leads to a slow metabolism. Of course, you have to be eating the right things; otherwise, the metabolism boost is negated by the weighty consequences (literally) of nutrient-poor food.

The key is quality, not quantity, because *calorie counting is not effective*. What *is* effective is knowing how our bodies use the different food groups. That way, you can make informed decisions about how to fuel your body optimally. You won't need to rely on any diet program or one-hundred-calorie marketing label. You won't need to count calories religiously or buy into expensive weight-loss programs that compose meals for you. Armed with the knowledge of how food biologically breaks down in the body, you can be creative and design your own meals and snacks. "What kind of protein do I want today? There aren't any healthy fats in this meal. Maybe I should add some avocado …"

How liberating! You won't ever again need to take someone else's word for it. You will be able to sort through all the diet crazes and contradictory weight-loss tips for yourself.

Let's put the reins back into your hands, where they should have been all along.

The Thermic Effect of Food (and Why It Matters)

Measuring the thermic effect of food (TEF) is different from measuring a calorie.[1] While calories measure how food breaks down in a laboratory setting, the TEF measures how food breaks down in a living, breathing human body, making it a much more relevant metric for assessing food quality. This isn't like golf where the lower the score, the better. We want as high of a TEF as possible, because that means the body is burning more calories as it extracts energy from the food. A diet of cheesecake and cookies has a low TEF. A diet of lean meat and vegetables has a high TEF.

About 10 percent of your overall caloric intake is burned off as the thermic effect of food, but you can increase or decrease this percentage depending on what you eat. For example, protein has a significantly higher TEF than either carbohydrates or fats; the body burns off about 25 percent of protein calories when turning it into either energy or body structure.[2] So technically, when counting ingested protein calories, you could knock off 25 to 30 percent because of its high burn rate. But remember, we're giving up the whole misleading calorie-counting thing altogether, so this is purely hypothetical, of course.

What happens to the other 90% of your total caloric intake? Well, 25 percent of it is spent on providing fuel to support your activity level. But you can positively affect this, too. By increasing your aerobic activity, you will increase lean muscle mass over time. Since a greater muscle mass demands more tissue oxygenation, thin, muscular bodies burn more calories than compact, flabby bodies. Even at rest, one pound of muscle burns about three times as much energy as a pound of body fat. That means that leaner people can eat more than people with more fat on their bodies, even without physical activity.[3] However unfair that is, it's a biological fact, and thus, it's another reason to strive to be thin. Body shape greatly affects the way fuel is conserved or burned.

The other 65 percent of your total caloric intake goes toward simply keeping you alive. This is the portion that dictates the speed of your metabolism along with how healthy you look and feel. Here's why it's so important to understand this concept. When your metabolic rate is high, your body will fizz and sparkle with productive energy. You'll experience an improved mood and nice skin, nails, and hair; your brain will be working optimally; and you'll be able to perform at your peak level. It's as if you are driving along a windy road at night, and finally someone turns the brights on.

Below, you'll find a list of ways to boost your metabolism. I'll expand on many of these principles in later chapters (hold tight!), but this list is here as an easy and comprehensive guide for your future reference.

Secrets to a Faster Metabolism

- Choose foods with a high TEF. Sources of lean protein, vegetables and nuts are the perfect examples. In fact, one study indicated that eating nuts boosts resting metabolism (when you're not even doing anything!) by 11 percent![4]

- Eat plenty of fiber. Complex carbohydrates have a higher TEF because sifting through fiber requires more energy. Make that body of yours work for its calories.

- Stay hydrated. Have you ever noticed how you become tired and lethargic when you're hot and thirsty? That's because dehydration lowers your metabolism as your body shuts down so that it doesn't perspire or waste valuable energy.[4] Furthermore, if you drink cold water, your body has to work like a hot water heater to bring it up to body temperature, expending energy in the process.

- Reduce stress and get adequate sleep. In a high-stress, exhausted state, the body secretes cortisol, which helps deposit belly fat.

- Maintain muscle tone. Muscle burns more calories than fat.

- Protect your gut's health with probiotics so that it can do its job efficiently and effectively.

- Never rely on sugar for energy. Sugar ingestion prevents the release of the very proteins that help break down fat stores.

- Eat superfoods (Refer to Chapter 9). Superfoods contain the biological ingredients that your body requires to run optimally. Without vitamins, cofactors (necessary for chemical reactions in the body) and protein, we're like bread without yeast: lifeless, dull and flat.

- If your metabolism seems especially slow, ask your doctor to run thyroid function tests. (The thyroid is in charge of regulating metabolism and body temperature).

- Take in some iodized salt every day. Iodine deficiency is the number one cause of hypothyroidism.[5] While you don't need to go overboard with the salt, cutting it out of your diet deprives your body of necessary nutrients and slows your metabolism.

- Avoid protein deficiency and patterns of semi-starvation/dieting like the plague. They lay the groundwork for thyroid malfunction and metabolic collapse.

- Understand the principles of how our bodies use food. Let this be your guide for life.

The Physiology of How Our Bodies Use Food

Put down your smartphone, and stop daydreaming; you're about to read some world-changing, mind-blowing, earth-shattering stuff!

You may not know it, but in your very hands lies a chart that is enough to throw everything that we once thought we knew about the food pyramid and balanced nutrition *out the window*!

This chart, from the Science of Health Index website, is the perfect evidentiary support for the type of diet I advocate. It shows exactly how our bodies use food from all three of the food categories. And it demonstrates how vital it is to evaluate food based on its function, not based on calories. As you carefully examine it, pay close attention to which foods are used for energy and which foods get stored as fat.[6]

Type of food	% used to fuel its own digestion	% used in body structure and processes	% eliminated as waste	% stored as body fat (not used as energy)	% used as energy (not stored as body fat)
Animal-based protein	60–70%	30–40%	5%	0%	0–100%
Natural oils and fats	40%	30–60%	5%	0–5%	as much as 50%
Nuts/seeds	45%	20%	10%	10%	15%
Grains	25%	10%	10%	50%	5%
Green, leafy vegetables	40%	5%	55%	0%	0%
Fruit	30%	5%	20% and 15%	45–50%	0%

Key things to note:

- Fifty percent of starchy carbohydrates are stored as body fat.
- Zero percent of protein is stored as body fat.
- Zero to ten percent of healthy fats are stored as body fat.
- Healthy fats and proteins are the most necessary for body structure and processes.
- Carbohydrates require the least amount of energy to digest (burn the fewest calories).
- Contrary to popular belief, starchy carbohydrates are not our main supply of energy! They provide us with a long-term energy source: body fat.

In order to understand why these facts are true, we're going to examine each of the three food groups—protein, fats, and carbohydrates—in a bit more detail. I promise to keep it as brief as possible, but we must understand this information in order to achieve a lifelong weight management regimen.

Protein

Protein should be your new BFF. It is the athlete's greatest friend, the dieter's companion, and the go-to food for anyone who wants satiety and energy. Moreover, it's what our bodies are made up of.

Researchers at the Harvard T.H. Chan School of Public Health summed it up this way:

> Take away the water and about 75% of your weight is protein ... It's in muscle, bone, skin, hair, and virtually every other body part or tissue. It makes up the enzymes that power many chemical reactions and the hemoglobin that carries oxygen in your blood.
>
> At least 10,000 different proteins make you what you are and keep you that way. Twenty or so basic building blocks, called amino acids, provide the raw material for all proteins ... Because the body doesn't store amino acids, as it does fats or carbohydrates, it needs a daily supply of amino acids to make new protein.[7]

This last bit is key. Unlike fat and glucose, *protein does not turn into storage* (a.k.a. body fat).[8] So we absolutely need to consume protein regularly to maintain health.

Luckily, our bodies can make ten of the twenty amino acids that we need in order to function. But the rest is up to our diets.[9] A complete protein source is one that has the appropriate proportions of essential amino acids that we cannot personally manufacture.

All meat and animal products, including dairy, contain complete protein sources. Unfortunately, this is not true of proteins derived from plants, which creates a serious conundrum for vegans and vegetarians, who often end up falling short of their daily protein requirements. Of course, there are ways to supplement the diet. Beans have a relatively high protein content, for instance. Still, you'd need to eat about *one and a half cups of beans at* each *meal* to equal the amount of protein in a small (three-ounce) serving of chicken or beef. That's a lot of beans (and a lot of gas). Actually, even that wouldn't cut it; you'd still have to complete your protein intake with nuts, seeds, rice, or corn in order to get a full complement of essential amino acids.

I empathize with those who are horrified by the unethical treatment of farm-raised animals. It's true that many of our agricultural practices are abhorrent and need to change. Moreover, I have tremendous respect for people who are willing to change their lifestyle to stand up for something they believe in. But when it comes to weight management and obtaining a healthy diet, I have to admit that vegetarians (and especially vegans) face an uphill battle.

Let's look at what happens to the body if a diet is protein deficient.

Low availability of amino acids leads to less hemoglobin and red blood cell synthesis, which in turn makes it harder for the body to get oxygen to tissues. Energy level drops; endurance drops. Less oxygen availability also hurts the body's metabolism and causes it to burn fewer calories. So protein-deficient individuals struggle with tiredness, reduced physical activity, decreased lean body mass, and weight-management difficulties.

Extreme deficiency of protein (kwashiorkor) is most apparent in impoverished parts of the world. You have probably seen pictures of children in Africa with bloated bellies and skeletal arms and legs. That is the heartbreaking look of protein malnutrition. These poor people are plagued with muscle wasting, a weakened immune system, heart failure, and respiratory system failure.

All this is to say, please make sure you are taking in enough protein, especially if you are vegetarian or vegan. Every meal and snack should contain protein because it is vital for satiety (the feeling of fullness). A good rule of thumb (so that you don't have to count grams) is that one serving size of protein is about the size and weight of your palm.

Fats

What do fats do for us? Actually, the more appropriate question is: What *don't* fats do for us? Fatty acids are essential for signal transduction and transcription, for the structure of cell walls and tissue, for a healthy heart, for a healthy brain, and for clean, flexible arteries. Fats provide a smooth energy source that cuts sweet cravings and hunger pains. They promote healing throughout the body and decrease inflammation. Their role in skin health is extraordinary, and they can even heal problematic skin conditions. They contribute to healthy hair. They lead to less dandruff and best of all, less cellulite! (Yup, you heard me right—less cellulite. Yet another blow to the myth that fat in the mouth equals fat on the body).

Perhaps most important, at least from a psychiatric perspective, is the fact that *fats are antidepressants*. They have been linked to feelings of well-being! Without them, we don't think as well and we suffer from a poor outlook on life. Fat-free nutrition, over any prolonged period of time, causes weight gain, obsessions with food, lack of energy, and depression. Supposedly, the man who started the fat-free nutrition craze developed severe depression and committed suicide. *Ouch!*[10, 11, 12]

Fats sound pretty magical, right? But are all fats safe?

Decisively, no. But the kinds of fats that are safe and those that are dangerous might surprise you, because society has taught almost exactly the opposite of what is true for decades.

We all know that saturated fats (animal fats) taste good. Butter, bacon, and cheese are delicious! Yet in the past, saturated fats have been the recipients of a lot of bad press. Medical science journals previously claimed that these fats contributed to heart disease, strokes, and obesity. Our population has shunned meat products and dairy fats based on a progressive campaign that maligned these foods.

But here is the good news. Saturated fats are actually vital for optimal body functioning. These fats help maintain the integrity of cell membrane walls; they help transport necessary chemicals into the cells and toxins out. They help protect us from viruses, yeast, and some harmful gut bacteria by contributing to the health of the immune system. They facilitate the absorption of vitamins. And as if all of that's not enough, these fats aid in heart protection, bone strength, liver protection, and asthma prevention.[13, 14, 15]

Dr. Mann from Vanderbilt University went as far as to call the belief that coronary heart disease is caused by a diet rich in saturated fat and cholesterol "the greatest scientific deception of the century, and perhaps any century."[16] In fact, no saturated fats are found in aortic plaque.

Another type of fat that we really want to take in is the omega-3 fatty acid. Omega-3 fatty acids are *king* in the world of nutrition. Perhaps you've heard of them? They've almost become a health craze on their own; they're all over food advertisements lately. But that's a good thing, because without omega-3's in our diet, our brains simply don't work well. Breast milk, which is perfectly formulated to provide the best nutrition to support life and grow a healthy brain, is particularly rich in omega-3 fatty acids. That should be a telling sign.

Omega-3's and their counterpart, omega-6's, are types of polyunsaturated fats.[17] It is important to note that they are called "essential fatty acids" because our bodies cannot produce them on their own! We have to take them in through our food (similar to the "essential amino acids" we discussed earlier in regards to protein). Ideally, we should consume these two types of essential fatty acids in a perfect 1:1 ratio.

Back in the time when humans were hunter-gatherers, maintaining that ratio was easy! Without any understanding of the biological breakdown of their food, hunter-gatherers had a diet of vegetables, seeds, nuts, and wild, grazing game that provided that perfect balance between omega-3's and omega-6's. It was natural. How do you think Americans today are doing with that balance?

Our current ratio of omega-3s to omega-6s is 1:20.[18] What a huge difference! We eat twenty times less omega-3 fats than we used to! How did that happen? *Omega-3 fats are found in wild game, grass-fed cattle, wild-caught fish, nuts, seeds, and greens,* and over the years, our diets have become consistently less reliant on these foods. Instead, we've become more reliant on grains and manufactured foods, like vegetable oils, which supply the majority of our omega-6's (and a large amount of our calories). Our current diets have completely wrecked the proper balance of fats that our bodies need.

This is actually a really, really bad thing, because an improper balance of these essential fatty acids has been linked to all sorts of horrible health problems. While omega-3's decrease inflammation and the risk of cancer, an excess of omega-6's does just the opposite; it increases inflammation and the risk of cancer.[19] Furthermore, many scientists believe that the past century's rapid rise in diabetes, obesity, and heart disease is due to the imbalance of fats in modern diets, along with the consumption of trans fats.[20]

Omega-3's are so vital to our neurologic health that deficiencies are currently being connected to ADHD, learning disabilities, Alzheimer's disease, inflammatory disorders, and many psychiatric disorders. If you are after a healthy body and lifestyle, you need to restore the proper balance of these essential fatty acids.

Okay. So replace omega-6 consumption with sources of saturated fats and omega-3 fats. Anything else?

Yes, one more thing. The fats that we should absolutely flee from like a cat flees from water are trans fats.

You see, it all comes down to their molecular structure. In saturated fats (animal fats), all of the carbon bonds have a hydrogen atom attached, which makes them chemically quite stable. That's really, really important because chemically *un*stable fats oxidize with exposure to heat or light (during cooking or even while sitting in the grocery store, in your kitchen, or in your body!) and can easily turn rancid. In order to neutralize this oxidation, the body must use up its store of antioxidants. The bottom line is that this oxidation process causes cell mutation, as seen with cancer, and inflammation, the source of most of the worst illnesses plaguing our society.

Guess which fats are chemically unstable—trans fats and omega-6 fatty acids. These are the types of fat that can lead to oxidation and diseased states.

Phew. I just threw a lot of information at you. But the bottom line is this: say *yes* to omega-3's, saturated fats, and monounsaturated fats. Say *no* to omega-6's and trans fats.[20] How do we keep track of that in our diets?[21]

Healthy Fat Sources	Fat Type(s)	Unhealthy Fat Sources	Fat Type(s)	Where It Hides
Coconut oil	Saturated fat, medium-chain fatty acids (produce energy instead of body fat and arterial plaque)	Margarine, shortening, any fake butter products	Trans fat	Sauces, salad dressings, fried foods
Grass-fed meat	Saturated fat, omega-3's	Corn/grain/soy-fed meat	omega-6's, saturated fat	American meats, unless otherwise specified
Eggs	Saturated fat, omega-3's	"Vegetable" oil, soybean oil, peanut oil, corn oil, safflower oil, palm oil, canola oil, cottonseed oil	omega-6's, trans fats produced during refining/manufacturing	Fried foods, manufactured/packaged snack products (chips, crackers), fast foods, condiments, sauces
Avocados, avocado oil, olives, olive oil	monounsaturated fats	Sunflower oil	As high as 70% omega-6's[23]	Artificial cheeses, roasted nuts
Pastured, grass-fed butter and cheese	Omega-3's, saturated fat			
Fish, fish oil (wild-caught, not farm raised)	Omega-3's			

Healthy Fat Sources	Fat Type(s)	Unhealthy Fat Sources	Fat Type(s)	Where It Hides
Flaxseed oil, ground flaxseed meal, chia seeds, walnut oil, macadamia nut oil	Extremely high in omega-3's, monounsaturated fat			
Nuts and seeds (*not* roasted in vegetable oil)	Omega-3's, monounsaturated fat			
Organic whole milk and cream	Saturated fat, omega-3's			

Luckily, the list of healthy fats is long and diverse, whereas the unhealthy fats are relatively easy to remember. Many of them come from vegetable oil and its many offshoots: canola oil, sunflower, safflower, soybean oil, and so on. These oils are typically in what I call *tame food* (as opposed to wild, natural food), which includes chips, cookies, crackers, fried fish/chicken, french fries, baking mixes (cake, cupcakes, etc.), manufactured bars (even the ones that use "health food" advertisements), cereal, bakery products, salad dressings, condiments, sauces, and the list goes on. Try finding a packaged or processed food not loaded with soy or corn oil and not dripping in unhealthy omega-6 fats. It's a challenge!

So is it worth it? Is it really that important for us to pay attention to the kinds of fats we're taking in?

Just remember your cell membranes are only as healthy as the fats you ingest. When you eat the wrong foods, you are ruining your cell wall membranes. They become damaged and rigid. Communication between cells becomes impaired, and the risk of arthritis, strokes, and heart disease increases. Pretty disastrous scenario, if you ask me.[24] I hope, though, your cell membranes aren't too rigid and impaired to be restored by changed eating patterns.

When deciding which oils to cook with, it's important to choose fats with high "smoke points," meaning fats that don't go rancid easily when they're heated up.[25] The best ones to cook with seem to be coconut oil and butter, because they do not oxidize easily or go rancid at high temperatures.[26] The science regarding which oils are safest to cook with is admittedly still evolving, so we'll have to keep our eyes and ears open in the future. Overall, it's safer to boil, bake, steam, or grill foods rather than fry them if you want to avoid messing up the chemical structure of your cooking oil.[27]

Carbohydrates

There's so much to say about how our bodies break down carbohydrates that we're actually going to devote the entire next chapter to this subject.

For now, I want to look at our society's emphasis on eating *heart-healthy* whole grains. Are they as good for you as the oatmeal, granola, and cereal bar commercials propose? Aren't multigrain, whole wheat, and whole grain products like bread and rice loaded with nutrients and fiber?

Unfortunately, grains are not the heart-friendly, healthy, ideal staples of our diet that many sources say they are. I will highlight three different harmful substances found in grains as evidence: phytic acid, lectin, and gluten.[28, 29]

Phytic acid is a mineral blocker; it prevents the absorption of nutrients, including calcium, iron, magnesium, copper, and zinc. Consequently, it is a major contributor to the huge increase in cases of osteoporosis we have seen in the past century. Phytic acid is found in the bran of all grains.

Lectin is a sugar-binding protein. In plants, it acts as a natural pesticide, fending off bugs and animals. When humans consume lectin, it prevents nutrient absorption, increases inflammation, and eventually leads to a host of diseases—cancer, diabetes, obesity, and heart disease, to name a few. It acts a lot like gluten, in fact.

Gluten

I bet you've heard of this substance before. The increasing number of people who are allergic or intolerant to gluten has led to a growing market for gluten-free products and even a gluten-free diet craze that has nothing to do with allergies. This may come as a surprise, but going gluten-free *for the sake of weight loss* is not effective. Gluten-free brownies, cookies, bread, and pasta are refined carbohydrates that turn into sugar in your body just as much as their gluten-full counterparts. Nevertheless, the fact that gluten causes so many people health problems begs the question: Is there something about this protein that is inherently detrimental, something that everyone should avoid?

In fact, yes. Gluten can prevent nutrient absorption and ultimately lead to diseased states because it causes something called *leaky-gut syndrome*.[30] What happens is that gluten irritates the cells in the intestinal walls, which then become inflamed and more permeable than they are supposed to be. As a result, tiny bits of food leak into the bloodstream, wreaking havoc in the GI tract and increasing inflammation all over the body. This is why gluten contributes to a whole slew of health problems in the long run, not just allergies[31]—to name a few: arthritis, autoimmune diseases, diabetes, cancer, acne, heart disease, and even mental illnesses, such as depression and schizophrenia.[32, 33] Some studies show evidence that infertility, obesity, and autism should be included in this list as well.[34, 35, 36]

Sadly celiac disease, or wheat/gluten intolerance, often goes undiagnosed for years or even a lifetime with devastating effects on the individual. The University of Chicago Celiac Disease Center tells us that undiagnosed celiac disease increases the risk of premature death by *four times* because of the large number of illnesses it can cause![37]

Why do you think it is that gluten only recently became a "thing" that we talk about? Is it because we are only now becoming aware of a health issue that has always been prevalent? Or have gluten intolerances and allergies really increased in frequency over the last few decades?

A study using fifty-year-old frozen blood samples from the Warren Air Force base in Cheyenne, Wyoming, gives us clear answers to these questions. The researchers, from the Mayo Clinic and the University of Minnesota, found that gluten intolerance is *four times* as common today as it was in the 1950s.[38] So it isn't simply increased awareness and detection; the ailment really has increased. And the change has everything to do with the evolution of the kind and amount of wheat that we eat.

You see, *gluten* was appropriately named after the Latin word for "glue"; it is a sticky substance that gives baked goods their appetizing texture.[39] (Less appetizing is the glue-like, constipating lump it becomes in your digestive system, but that's another story). That desirable characteristic has led to a dramatic increase in the amount of gluten in modern strains of wheat—Thank you, modern technology—and makes our refined, processed flours, even the ones in the supposedly heart-healthy whole grain products, completely different than the rough grains our ancestors ate.[40] That is the reason it seems like gluten allergies are an invention of the day, because they are, just as much as techno music and smartphones. They're part of our society's invention of the highly processed, carbohydrate-dense modern diet.

Foods with mucus-like properties (i.e., flaxseed meal, chia seeds, okra, and edible seaweeds) have been shown to combat the disease-causing processes of digesting gluten, phytic acid, and lectin.[41, 42] Yet these are hardly staples of the American diet, wouldn't you say?

Ultimately, our best hope of warding off these disease-producing processes is to limit our intake of the very starches that *are* staples of the all-American diet, even the multigrain and whole wheat products that boast of an endless list of health benefits. *For a good laugh, check out The Appendix of this book. The cofounders of South Park created a hilarious episode called "Gluten Free Ebola" after going on a gluten-free diet themselves, and I couldn't help but include an excerpt from the script. The parody of the USDA's changing nutritional guidelines and the gluten-free craze was just too good to pass up …*

Summary
How Our Bodies Use Food

- Because calories are *not* all equivalent, calorie counting is *not* an effective means of weight control.

- The laboratory measurement of a calorie does not take into account the thermal effect of food (TEF) or how calories from various food groups affect metabolism differently.

- Maximizing metabolism is crucial for long-term weight management. In order to do so, be sure to…

  - Stay hydrated (dehydration slows metabolism)
  - Eat foods with a high TEF. Remember:
    - Proteins and fats have a higher TEF than carbohydrates (i.e., nuts increase metabolism by up to 11 percent).
    - Complex carbohydrates have a higher TEF than simple carbohydrates (i.e., lentils versus white potatoes).
  - Exercise moderately. Lean muscle burns more calories than fat.
  - Reduce stress and get adequate sleep.
  - Protect gut health by taking in probiotics through supplements or food sources.
  - Eat superfoods, not sugar-foods.
  - Avoid reaching a point of starvation, whether through dieting or skipping meals. Dieting and semistarvation slow down metabolism.

- Key things to note about how our bodies use food:

  - Fifty percent of starchy carbohydrates are stored as body fat.
  - Zero percent of protein is stored as body fat.
  - Zero to ten percent of healthy fats are stored as body fat.

- Carbohydrates require the least amount of energy to digest (you burn the fewest calories breaking them down).

- Contrary to popular belief, starchy carbohydrates are not the best source of energy! What they provide us with is a long-term energy source—body fat.

- We cannot live without consuming adequate amounts of proteins since they are the building blocks of life.

- As our satiety factor, fats help us feel full. They also boost mood, support brain function, and maintain our bodies' youth and vivacity.

- The true types of detrimental fats are trans fats and vegetable oils.

- Our society eats about twenty times the amount of omega-6 fats as it should, which puts us at risk for cancer, heart disease, obesity, and diabetes.

- Omega-6's are easily oxidized with light or heat exposure—whether on a grocery store shelf, during cooking, or in our bodies. And this oxidization depletes our bodies of *antioxidants*, causing numerous deficiencies along with inflammation and cell mutation, which are the beginnings of many disease states.

- In order to restore the proper balance of fats in our diets, we need to increase our consumption of omega-3's.

- Our society's fear of saturated fats is misguided. Because they are stable under heat, they do not oxidize easily and create free radicals in the body.

- At this point, the most stable fats to cook with are coconut oil and butter. Conflicting scientific findings on other oils means we should stay tuned for further research.

- Grains should not be considered the heart-healthy staples that government recommendations and ad campaigns hype them up to be.

- Grains contain phytic acid, lectin, and gluten—three harmful substances that interfere with nutrient absorption. They also cause inflammation and contribute to a whole host of diseases, like cancer, diabetes, heart disease, osteoporosis, inflammatory bowel conditions, autoimmune disorders, diabetes, and more.

- Going gluten-free does not make people lose weight. Gluten-free products can be just as successful as their gluten-full counterparts at providing the refined sugar and starchy carbohydrates that cause fat storage.

- Foods with mucous-like properties, including flaxseed, chia seeds, okra, and edible seaweeds, have the ability to combat some of the disease-causing processes initiated by the toxins in grains.

~ 5 ~

The Glycemic Index

In the last chapter, I promised I would finish talking about how our bodies break down carbohydrates. Am I getting too detailed? How much of this is really necessary to understand in order to maintain a lower weight and a healthy body?

Only what I've included here. I promise; I won't give you superfluous scientific information. Nevertheless, some knowledge of nutritional science is vital to your ability to make informed decisions about what you eat and buy. I don't want to simply give you a list of dos and don'ts or good foods and bad foods. You're smarter than that. You deserve to live a life ungoverned by dietary rules, calorie counting, or punitive regimens. You deserve to be equipped with wisdom and discernment so you can cook, eat, and live creatively and richly.

A Spoonful of Sugar

The first thing you need to know is that carbohydrates are broken down into glucose and thus raise your blood sugar level. Too high of blood sugar leads to hyperglycemia and, in the long run, diabetes. Thankfully, we have an organ whose sole job is to prevent this from happening: the pancreas.

When you eat carbohydrates, the pancreas secretes the hormone insulin in order to lower your blood sugar again. Insulin takes whatever glucose isn't needed for immediate energy and tucks it away as fat.[1] Moreover, insulin actually prevents existing fat from being broken down, too! Obviously, no one likes the guy whose job is to create and maintain body fat. But believe me, it's a lot better than the alternative. Without insulin, we'd continue to have an excess of sugar in the blood, and while sweet blood sounds benign, the problems that stem from an elevated sugar level are so extensive that they impact every organ of the body. Excess sugar injures the walls of the small blood vessels that nourish the nerves, eyes, kidneys, skin, brain, and virtually every other organ. Eventually, tissue damage occurs, vision is impaired, wounds don't heal, kidneys fail... Our bodies simply cannot handle the effects of a lifetime of too many carbohydrates. So thank goodness for the pancreas and insulin!

The problem is that the pancreas can only take so much before it burns out, especially since it has other things to worry about besides insulin deployment. In fact, only 1 percent of the pancreas is devoted to producing insulin. Ninety-nine percent of the pancreas is actually devoted to processing protein and natural fats.[2] And what happens when the pancreas burns out?

Diabetes is what happens. Faaantastic.

Too many people today suffer with this very serious illness. The American Diabetes Association reports that in 2012, 29.1 million Americans had diabetes. That's almost one out of every ten people.[3] Worse still, nearly one in four adolescents are either on the verge of developing diabetes or already suffer with it![4]

Shhhhhhhh! Do you hear that? If you listen really closely, you can just about make it out. Yup, your pancreas is begging you, "Please pay attention to your carbohydrate intake!"

What Is the Glycemic Index, and Why Should We Care?

We always want to avoid extremes when eating. So rather than vowing to never put another carbohydrate to our lips, let's look at ways we can be smart about our carbohydrate intake to keep our pancreas (and our body!) healthy. One fantastic way to do this is by understanding the glycemic index of the food you eat.

The glycemic index (GI) is essentially the body's sweetness indicator for foods. Its number value reflects how quickly and to what extent your blood sugar level will rise after consuming a food or beverage. On a scale from 0 to 100, high-glycemic-indexed carbohydrates break down quickly and call for a big insulin response. Low-GI carbs, on the other hand, are more complex and thus break down more slowly and do not cause a spike in blood sugar levels. *So by sticking with low-GI carbs, you will avoid huge insulin responses that create and maintain fat stores.*

Why do I emphasize carbohydrates? Well, protein and fats would all fall in the lowest GI category because they do not significantly raise your blood sugar. (Remember from last chapter: protein and fat do not get turned into storage material).[5]

Please take a few minutes to examine the Glycemic Index Chart on the following page. What patterns do you notice? Does nutrition quality increase or decrease as you move from left to right?

	Extra-Low GI (0–15)	Low GI (15–35)	Medium GI (35–60)	High GI (60–100)
Vegetables and Root Vegetables	broccoli, cabbage, mushrooms, onions, lettuce **10**		green peas, carrots **48**	beets **69**
	cauliflower, spinach, asparagus, peppers, green beans, celery **15**		sweet potato, corn **55**	baked potato **93** parsnips **97**
Fruits	tomato **15**	cherries **22**	apple, pear, plum **38–39**	dried figs/ raisins **60**
		grapefruit **25**	orange **45**	melon/ cantaloupe **65**
		berries **32**	kiwi **52** banana, mango, grapes **55**	pineapple **66**
			fruit juices **50–60**	watermelon **72**
Breads, Grains		pearled barley **30**	multigrain bread **48**	rye bread **64** wholemeal bread **69**
			oatmeal **52**	Special K, Muesli **69**
			quinoa, brown rice **53** wild rice **57**	white rice **70** white bread **71** bagel **72**
			pasta **55**	cheerios, crackers **74**
			granola **56**	doughnut **76** rice cakes **77**
			popcorn, potato chips **58**	cornflakes, pretzels **83**

	Extra-Low GI (0–15)	Low GI (15–35)	Medium GI (35–60)	High GI (60–100)
				baguette **91**
Beans	hummus **10**	lentils **30** chickpeas **33**	pinto beans **39** baked beans **48**	broad beans **79**
Dairy	whole milk yogurt **14**	whole milk **22** fat-free yogurt **30** skimmed milk **32**		ice cream **61**
Other	nuts **10**	dark chocolate (75% + cocoa) **<30**	milk chocolate **48–60** power bar **58**	honey **62** tofu frozen desert **115**

Let's take a closer look at some of the specifics from the chart.[6] Are you surprised by the placement of any foods? How about watermelon? Did you notice that it has a higher GI than ice cream? At a very high 91 and 93, baguettes and baked potatoes look more like treats than staples, right? And eating white rice doesn't look all that different from indulging in a doughnut. Of course, watermelon, dates, and potatoes offer nutritional value that doughnuts and pretzels do not. Still, their sugar content is so high that they should only be eaten in moderation.

Pay particular attention to everything on the far left. Nonstarchy vegetables are all in this category of highest-quality carbs. These are your *free* foods: leafy greens, green beans, radishes, peppers, celery, cucumbers, cauliflower, broccoli, zucchini, squash, asparagus, brussels sprouts, and so on. You never have to worry about overeating these colorful carbs. In contrast, the starchier vegetables and grains, like corn, rice, potatoes, cooked carrots, and bakery products, bump up your glycemic load rather quickly. Consequently, eat few of these items and keep serving sizes small.

Lower-GI foods are also typically the ones with more fiber, making them both filling and particularly nutritious. Fiber is the only carbohydrate that isn't broken down into sugar! And both types, soluble and insoluble fiber, do some amazing things for the body.

Soluble fiber is so named because it dissolves in water. It binds to the really bad fat molecules, called LDLs, and carries them out as waste! This is why eating fiber reduces heart disease and our risk for strokes. In addition, this type of fiber provides the bulk that keeps us feeling full. *Sources include oat bran, flaxseed, apples, oranges, celery, carrots, barley, and dried legumes, such as peas and lentils.*

Insoluble fiber does not dissolve in water. This type of fiber helps food move through the gut efficiently—and prevents constipation. And that's always a good thing. *Sources include whole grains and vegetables, seeds, nuts, barley, whole wheat, broccoli, cabbage, onions, tomatoes, green beans, cucumbers, fruit, root vegetable skins, and corn bran.*[7, 8]

Fiber is extremely important for weight management, fullness, blood sugar control, and lipid balance. Most people take in around fifteen grams of fiber or less each day, falling far short of the desired twenty to thirty grams per day. The widespread deficiency is largely due to the way our food is now produced. We put raw carbohydrate ingredients through a food Laundromat. We strip, scrub, and bleach every rough edge off of grains until they are sparkling white and tasteless. Then we add corn syrup/sugar and fat to flour and feed this paste to people in many forms: white bread, cake, scones, animal crackers, cookies, cinnamon rolls, pancakes, battered fried foods, and so on. This is not the way carbohydrates were meant to be eaten. In nature, they come wrapped in fiber. Let's leave them that way.

It's also important to know that quantity matters as well as quality. Since insulin is secreted in proportion to the *net amount of sugar* in the blood, the body responds the same way whether the sugar comes from a small amount of very sugary foods (carbs with a high GI) or a larger amount of less sugary foods (carbs with a low GI). Put simply, the greater the quantity of carbohydrates, whether they're brownies or blueberries, the more your blood sugar will rise and the more insulin is secreted. *So keep the GI of the carbohydrates in your diet* and *the amount you're eating down.*

Until you get the hang of the glycemic index chart, you might need to keep one handy so you can refer to it as you need. But luckily, you unknowingly carry a portable glycemic index with you wherever you go—your mouth and eyes. When you don't know a food's glycemic index, these two sensory organs can usually give you clues. Ask yourself the following questions:

Does this food taste sweet? What type of sugar does it contain? Is it table sugar? Is it fruit sugar, honey, corn syrup, saccharin, or Stevia? Table sugar (sucrose) has a much higher GI than fructose (the sugar found in fruit), so that's a very important question to ask. Also, concentrated, processed, and refined sugars will most likely trigger the largest insulin response. Obviously, the best choice is to keep it natural; sugar encased in fiber and fructose comes in a fibrous fruit.

Here's how your eyes can be of help. White foods tend to have a higher glycemic index than *naturally* colorful foods. (Note the emphasis on *naturally*—I did not just give you my blessing to go "taste the rainbow" with a bag of Skittles). For example, the glycemic index of a white russet potato or white rice is nearly twice that of the orange sweet potato. A bit counterintuitive, isn't it? You'd think *sweet* potatoes would have a higher GI. But they follow the naturally colorful rule. Also, refined foods stripped of fiber will have higher glycemic indexes. Hence, white rice has a slightly higher GI than whole grain, brown rice.

Still, some studying of the actual chart is very useful because our eyes and mouth can be deceived. For instance, you might not guess that berries have a much lower GI than bananas, melon, and grapes, all of which lead to larger insulin spikes.

You might be wondering, *How important is this, really? Will it honestly affect me that much if I try to adhere to a low-GI, high-fiber diet?*

To answer, here's a powerful fact. People who eat high-GI foods for breakfast tend to eat about 53 percent more food later in the day than people who eat a low-GI breakfast.[9] The more simple, high-GI carbohydrates we eat, the more we crave.

Why? Because of a simple maxim: what goes up must come down. Think about the cycle. You eat a large carbohydrate load, and your blood sugar spikes. Then insulin kicks in and tucks the glucose away (probably onto your belly or thighs), which causes the blood sugar to drop again. It is this drop that causes fatigue, possible shakiness, and even irritability and *more hunger.* Taking in more carbohydrates will solve the problem! (Note the sarcasm dripping off the page.)

People often choose to eat hefty meals of carbohydrates with the misconception that this will tide them over longer. Am I right? Eat a huge plate of pasta for lunch to last you all afternoon. Sounds logical. But now you know; the more carbs you eat, the bigger the drop you'll feel (in energy, mood, and satiation), and you'll just want to eat again sooner rather than later.[10, 11]

It's important to note that the rate of this blood sugar drop is related to the rate that the food breaks down in the body. In other words, the unpleasant bottoming-out feeling will be much worse with a big load of fiberless, high-GI foods (perhaps a few pastries, doughnuts, or a sugary muffin) than with a balanced meal of a few fiber-filled carbs, protein, and healthy fats.[12, 13]

Blood Sugar Response to Carbs

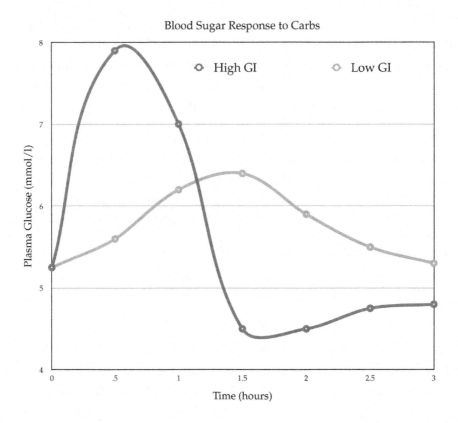

The terrible roller-coaster ride with bursts of insulin every couple of hours leads to mood swings and hypoglycemic episodes. Yet we don't credit those negative side effects to our delicious, refined carbohydrates. Instead, we only associate them with the initial burst of energy and happiness—the addictive sugar high.

Sugar Addicts

This must be an exaggeration, right? Can food actually be biologically or psychologically addictive in the same way that drugs or alcohol can be?

With brief synopses of five startling studies, I believe I can convince you of the affirmative.[14] Hang on to your hat.

1. At Princeton University, psychologists tried to determine whether or not lab rats could become addicted to a 10 percent sugar solution (*the quantity seen in most soft drinks!*). Turns out, they can. When rats were given 24/7 access to the sugar-water solution, they chose to drink in all their calories and stopped eating altogether. Crazier yet, when the sugar formula was taken away from them, they demonstrated withdrawal symptoms, like shakiness, anxiety, and even neurochemical changes in the brain. One more note on this study—when the rats were given water sweetened with high fructose corn syrup instead of sugar, they became obese *as well as* addicted. That's just dandy. After all, American manufacturers currently use corn syrup to sweeten the majority of our food and drink products.

2. In 2010, scientists wanted to determine how rats act when given a choice between healthy and unhealthy food. The first of two groups of rats was given access to nutritious food all day long and to junk food for only one hour out of the day. Guess what. The scientists noticed that the rats ignored the healthy food all day long, starving themselves in preparation for the one-hour junk food allotment. When that hour came, they binge-ate the rich, fattening food (cheesecake, bacon, frosted cake, cookies, etc.). The second group of rats had both kinds of food available to them all day long. These rats became huge. Not only did they choose the rich foods over the healthy foods, but they also chose to keep eating them all day long, gorging themselves to the point of obesity. Moreover, the high sugar/fat food elicited the same kind of response in the rat brains' reward centers as cocaine.[15]

3. Another 2010 study taught us that these same reward centers can't get as excited about sweets if people consume a lot of them on a regular basis. These "happy places" of the brain become tolerant to milkshakes much like a drug addict becomes tolerant to drugs. Higher and higher doses of rich food become necessary for brain excitement to occur. Over time, people become desensitized to sweets.

4. Another study looked at women's brain patterns while under the influence of sweets. Women drinking milkshakes showed brain patterns that looked like an alcoholic's brain when anticipating a drink.

5. A 2007 study from the University of Bordeaux in France found that rats prefer water that's been sweetened with either sugar or saccharin (a calorie-free sweetener) to cocaine. Even if they had been cocaine addicts previously!

Interestingly, these studies were highlighted in an article titled, "Fatty Foods Addictive as Cocaine."[16] Do you see the problem with that title? What was the real addictive substance in each of these studies? Was it fat? Or was it sugar? Look back through each of them if you're not sure. Yup, your eyes aren't deceiving you. There aren't any studies showing rats getting addicted to avocados or olive oil. Sugar, not fat, was the universal addictive substance in these studies. Whether living creatures are put on high-sugar diets or high-sugar/high-fat diets, their brains build up a tolerance and require more and more of their drug to feed their addiction to sweetness.

The Truth about Artificial Sweeteners

One last question before I give you an information overdose: Why don't we just use artificial sweeteners to satisfy our sweet tooth while avoiding the calories?

I found conflicting information on this topic, but the evidence thus far indicates that it's not a good idea. While in the laboratory we find that aspartame, saccharin, and Splenda have no caloric value, other interesting reactions are happening in our bodies that we cannot assess in a lab. What we *do* know is that diet-soda drinkers increase their risk of developing metabolic syndrome[17] more so than regular-soda drinkers! Why is that a big deal? Metabolic syndrome describes a package of weight-related health problems that is best measured by the amount of central body fat that people have. Basically, this implies that diet-soda drinkers are gaining belly fat faster than non-diet-soda drinkers!

I bet you're skeptical about that last statement, and I don't blame you. Let's see if I can convince you with a bit more evidence ...

Sharon Fowler, MPH, and colleagues from the Texas Health Science Center found that diet-soda drinkers gain more weight per year than sugar-sweetened soda drinkers. They reported, "There was a 41% increase in risk of being overweight for every can or bottle of diet soft drink consumed each day." Wow. These researchers also witnessed that rat pups that are fed with artificial sweeteners crave more calories than those that are fed real sugar.[18]

One theory even claims that low-calorie diet drinks stimulate our appetites. How could that be possible? Well, according to this theory, when someone drinks a diet soda, his or her body secretes enough insulin for the amount of sugar it *thinks* it's getting. So if a diet drink is sweet enough that the body expects 200 calories of sugar energy, but the drink doesn't deliver, the body tries to get those 200 calories from another source. It might, for instance, make you crave 200 calories of fries to go along with that diet soda.

All signs point to this: if diet soda is potentially *worse* for us than normal soda, we should probably stay away from artificial sweeteners.

It definitely makes sense for our bodies to secrete a lot of insulin in response to these artificial sweeteners. After all, if they fool our tongue, they may fool our other sensors also. Interestingly, some research suggests that we have gut taste receptors that also sense the sweetness of sweeteners and then, you guessed it, signal the pancreas to boost its insulin secretion. *So even though artificial sweeteners do not have caloric value, they may still be causing insulin secretion and thus, a tendency to put on fat.*

Glucagon—the Natural Diet Pill

You've heard a lot about how the pancreas uses insulin to bring down our blood sugar when it gets too high. But what happens when our blood sugar gets too low? Does the pancreas have an antidote for that too?

Glucagon, another pancreatic hormone, brings our blood sugar level *up* by breaking down existing energy reserves. In other words, glucagon breaks down fat. Sounds exactly like what everyone wants. How do we get more of *that*?

When we eat a protein-rich, low-carbohydrate meal, the pancreas releases more glucagon. Not surprisingly, the best way to decrease your body fat percentage is to eat a protein-rich, low-carb, low-GI diet. As you will recall from "Diets Gone Wild," this is one of the few known methods of altering your set point, or the weight around which your body naturally hovers.

So while drug companies have fooled us into buying their dangerous, addictive, and health-destroying diet pills, we've had the recipe for fat burning all along. It is *not* in a low-fat, whole-grain, carbohydrate-rich diet like we've been led to believe.

I'll say it one last time so you have no chance to miss the point: *The best way to decrease your body fat percentage is to eat a protein-rich, low-carb, low-GI diet.*

But remember when we lose weight very slowly (at the rate of one to two pounds per month), our bodies do not shut down as if they were in a state of semistarvation. Be patient!

In the end, it's your choice. If you choose to keep your body fat at a lower percentage, then learn to make desserts the rare treat that they're meant to be. The good news is when people are able to take sugar out of their diet for an extended period of time, they find that they become sensitive to the taste of sweetness again. It's like hitting the reset button on the body's overused and desensitized sugar receptors. Moreover, most people find that they don't even like candy and desserts like they used to. They start to taste fake, almost plastic-y. You'll see. You eventually realize that your body doesn't feel as good when you eat sweets, which, if you think about it, is the truth—the sugar addiction has just been masking it all along.

Long story short, it gets easier and easier to resist sweets over time. And you'll start to enjoy the nutritious food you eat more and more. You'll be able to fully appreciate the array of subtle, natural flavors that you missed before. And you can't fail to notice how much better your body feels, almost as if it were *natural* to eat *naturally* ... or something.

Summary
The Glycemic Index

- When you eat carbohydrates (which the body converts into glucose), the pancreas secretes the hormone insulin.

- Insulin takes whatever glucose isn't needed for immediate energy and tucks it away as fat. It even prevents existing fat from being broken down or burned off!

- When our pancreas burns out or when our organs develop a resistance to insulin, we suffer with diabetes and all the related health problems.

- Cutting down on carbohydrates will …

  - decrease the burden placed on an overworked pancreas

  - force the pancreas to secrete glucagon (instead of insulin), which makes the body break down its fat stores to create glucose

- The glycemic index (GI) is essentially the body's sweetness indicator for foods.

- By sticking with low GI carbs, we avoid huge insulin responses, mood swings, and hypoglycemia.

- Fiber is the only carbohydrate that isn't broken down into sugar. Both soluble and insoluble fiber are important for weight management, satiety (fullness), blood sugar control, and lipid (fat) balance.

- Since insulin is secreted in proportion to the *net amount of sugar* in the blood, quantity of carbohydrates matters just as much as quality.

- Large carbohydrate doses lead to a burst of insulin secretion and then a subsequent crash in blood sugar, a terrible roller-coaster ride that causes mood swings and hypoglycemic episodes.

- Even though artificial sweeteners do not have caloric value, they may still be causing insulin secretion and thus a tendency to put on fat.

- The best way to decrease your body fat percentage is to eat a protein-rich, low-carb, low-GI diet.

~ 6 ~

The X-Factor:
Xamining Xtreme Xercise

I'm sure you know many women and men who compulsively exercise as a weight-management technique. You know—those disciplined individuals who wake up at the crack of dawn to run five miles or spend an hour on the elliptical or bike as soon as they get off of work. Perhaps you are one of them! And we've already discussed how bulimic individuals can use punitive exercise as a way to purge after eating.

Society tells us that extreme exercise is necessary for weight management. Weight-loss programs and TV shows like *The Biggest Loser* include demanding, daily workouts in their weight-loss regimens. Magazines constantly highlight different celebrities' workout routines so you can get a bod like J-Lo, Beyoncé—you name it! And there are always new exercise crazes to join in on—spin classes, Pure Barre ("the fastest, most effective way to change your body"),[1] even pole dancing has become a hip way to get in shape.

Fitness clubs are scoring big-time as a result of these trends. Memberships have gone up from 32.8 million Americans in 2000 to 54.1 million Americans in 2014.[2] And that's saying nothing of people who work out at home or outside.

All this fitness commotion brings up a few pertinent questions: Does your quest for health have to include hours of intense exercise every week? How necessary is exercise for weight management? And is it possible to go too far?

To make sure we take a fact-based approach to answering these questions, I'll defer to some fascinating studies.

Dr. Timothy Church, the chair of Health Wisdom at the Pennington Biomedical Research Center in Louisiana, investigated how much and to what extent exercise facilitates weight loss.[3] To do this, he placed 464 women on one of four different exercise regimens. One group worked out for 1.2 hours per week, another group for 2.3 hours per week, another for 3.2 hours per week, and the last group was instructed not to alter their normal routine (lucky ducks). What's your prediction for which group lost the most weight after six months?

Trick question. There was actually no statistical difference in over-all weight loss. So it didn't matter whether the subjects exercised for over three hours or none at all!

Dr. Church attributes this phenomenon to compensation.[4] You see, after an intense workout, people naturally balance out their caloric expenditure by doing the following:

A. decreasing their activity level after the workout (becoming couch potatoes)
B. feeding an increased appetite through greater food intake (with bigger portions *and* more frequent consumption)
C. rewarding themselves with energy-dense, high-calorie foods

Because of these compensation mechanisms, Dr. Church concludes, "Calorie for calorie, it's easier to lose weight by dieting than by exercise."[5]

Part of the reason we overcompensate is because we tend to over-estimate caloric expenditure. We all want to think we're burning a million calories every time we run a mile when in reality, it's probably less than one hundred.

Meanwhile, we *under*estimate how many calories we're taking in. After all, a piece of coffee cake is only, what, like, fifty calories? Nice try. Dr. Susan Jebb, head of nutrition and health research at Medical Research Council sums it up with this: "You have to do an awful lot more exercise than most people realize. To burn off an extra 500 calories is typically an extra 2 hours of cycling. That takes care of about 2 doughnuts."[6] Can you believe it? Who wants to do 120 minutes of intense cycling just to eat their doughnuts?

In what is perhaps an even more powerful study, researchers from Children's Hospital Boston observed the effect of physical activity on the eating habits of 538 students for eighteen months. Their findings confirmed Dr. Church's work. When the participants in their study exercised, they ate as much as *ten to twenty times* more calories than they had burned off through their workout. They *over*compensated for the energy gap created through activity. In plain terms, exercising made them eat too much.[7]

Yeesh! So it definitely *is* possible to go overboard with exercising.

Interestingly, research also shows that excessive exercise may actually contribute to a deterioration of health. Since it leads to fatigue and muscle/joint aches, the body releases more stress hormones. That's a really bad thing because besides being a factor in many disease states, our primary stress hormone, cortisol, actually makes our bodies want to put on more belly fat![8, 9]

If this information is making you jump for joy because you think you never have to do crunches or run another mile, sorry to burst your bubble. I'm not advocating for *no exercise*. Exercise is still vital for healthy living. It only becomes detrimental when taken too far.

How far is too far?

According to Barry Braun, associate professor of kinesiology at the University of Massachusetts, evidence shows that "low-intensity ambulation" (i.e., walking) may help to burn calories "without triggering a caloric compensation effect" (without making you reach for a snack the moment you're done). In fact, in one experiment, Braun showed that simply standing instead of sitting uses up hundreds of calories more in a day *without increasing appetite hormones in the blood*.[10]

Emma John of the UK newspaper, the *Guardian*, correctly summed up the implications of these studies when she wrote: "The latest scientific findings from the US suggest that an intense workout in the gym is actually less effective than gentle exercise in terms of weight loss."[11]

If all this is true, why is that everyone nowadays thinks more is better when it comes to exercising with the goal of weight loss?

It all goes back to the 1960s when one individual made some far-reaching assumptions and—badabing badaboom—exercise became a cornerstone treatment for weight loss.

Here's how it happened. Back in 1953, a nutritionist named Jean Mayer noticed that fidgety babies and children *ate more* and *weighed less* than calm babies and children.[12] What's more, he saw the same trend hold true in high school: the thin adolescent girls in his studies ate several hundred calories more than the overweight girls. Searching for an explanation for this seeming paradox, he landed on the difference in physical activity between the two groups. Since the overweight girls spent roughly one-third as much time in physical activity as the thin girls, it seemed logical to conclude that their lack of exercise was the primary reason for their weight problems.

Dr. Jean Mayer went on to work for the Nixon, Ford, and Carter administrations.[13] During this time, he had a clear mission: to put exercise at the core of the physical education and weight-management dialogue in America. It is largely thanks to him that we emphasize the importance of workouts for weight management even today.

Why do I see this as a problem? Because Dr. Mayer made a huge assumption that led to the wrong conclusion, and it has influenced our society tremendously. He grouped all physically active people together as "people who exercise" and failed to make the crucial distinction between those who put themselves through grueling workouts and those who just naturally move around a lot. I highly doubt that the "fidgety" babies in his initial observations, those who ate more but stayed thinner, were making daily trips to SoulCycle, but according to his inferences, they might as well have been.

Correcting the Harmful Misperceptions: What Level of Exercise is Best for Weight Management?

In order to correct Dr. Mayer's mistake, let's clarify the difference between the two types of physically active people. First, there are those who expend almost their entire energy quota in one gigantic burst of activity and then spend the rest of the day wiped out. Just like Dr. Church found in the studies I mentioned above, after intense workouts, people compensate by moving less and even being less productive. It's only natural for them to crave time to rest and recover. These aerobic fiends often complain that they have bulky thighs or too much muscle, all the while refusing to blame it on the excessive exercising (and compensatory eating) that causes it.

Meanwhile, there are those tightly wired people who burn their calories steadily throughout the day; their metabolism is fired up from morning until night rather than for only one or two hours. Perhaps they do yoga or Pilates. On a summer day, they may go for a long walk, a hike, or a pleasant bike ride. They'll play tennis or go swimming or Rollerblading. Whatever they do, they are neither stationary nor involved in brutal fitness routines. Thus, they burn fat but don't get bulky or thick; they have just enough strength in their lean muscles.

While both groups benefit from physical activity, their energy expenditure is different and that leads to varying physiological consequences.

What about the mental health benefits of exercise, though? If not for weight maintenance, shouldn't we still engage in intense workouts for the positive psychological side effects? Actually, research shows that moderate exercise alone provides all the mental health benefits that come from physical activity.[14, 15] So more is better doesn't even apply in this regard.

How relieving it is to know that we don't have to whip ourselves into shape.[16] We can do it gently and intelligently.

Now that we know what kind of physical activity is best, let's look at what it actually does for us.

The Health Benefits of Physical Activity

Here are some of the myriad of ways that exercise benefits the body, mind, and spirit:

- improves psychological well-being (it's a mood-booster)
- reduces stress
- enhances mental clarity and acuity
- boosts metabolism
- supports strong immune system functioning
- improves skin/complexion
- helps regulate digestive system
- builds stamina, strengthens heart, lowers heart rate
- enhances work, recreation, and sport performance
- strengthens and maintains healthy muscles, bones, and joints[17]
- reduces the risk of premature death and the development of:
  - heart disease
  - high blood pressure
  - high cholesterol

- colds and flus
- cancer
- diabetes
- depression and anxiety[18]

As you can see, the benefits of exercise are incredible. Let me highlight and explain just a few important things from this list.

The reason exercise enhances mental acuity is because it increases blood flow, allowing more oxygen and nutrients to reach your brain. That's why being active actually allows you to think better! Similarly, better circulation delivers more nutrients to your skin, allowing it to produce more collagen (which keeps skin plump, taut, and youthful), and flushes out toxins. All this improves complexion and gives your skin a healthy glow.

Weight-bearing exercise in particular has the power to strengthen your bones as well as your muscles. Consequently, engaging in physical activity, while including vitamin D and calcium in your daily diet, is a great way to safeguard against osteoporosis.

There's also the amazing fact that exercise boosts metabolism. In "How Our Bodies Use Food," we learned that muscle burns more energy than fat, even when you're at rest. So much so that an additional five pounds of muscle causes your body to spend an extra 175–250 calories per day.[19] Since men have greater muscle mass than women typically, women should be doing something physical almost every day to enjoy the benefits of a lean but strong musculature.

By far the most important benefit of exercise, in my opinion, is the positive impact it has on mental health. As Elle Woods aptly pointed out in the classic 2001 film *Legally Blonde*, "Exercise gives you endorphins. Endorphins make you happy. Happy people just don't shoot their husbands. They just don't!"[20] Well, she was certainly right about one thing: levels of endorphins in the blood increase when you work out, which does have a mood-boosting effect. Actually, levels of the neurochemical serotonin rise in the brain as well. Since depression is associated with low levels of both endorphins and serotonin, this is incredible. And it makes sense, then, that physically active people lower their risk of depression by as much as 50 percent![21] No wonder physical activity can be an effective treatment for mood and anxiety disorders.

So what are you waiting for? Grab your running shoes, your tennis shoes, your ballet shoes, your bowling shoes, those weird barefoot shoes that have separate compartments for all your toes ... and exercise.

Exercise, but don't kill yourself. There's no need! Intense, hardcore workouts are ineffective and even counterproductive as a weight-loss technique.[22, 23, 24] Exercise moderately, with joy and enthusiasm.

Summary
The X-Factor: Xamining Xtreme Xercise

- After an intense workout, people naturally do the following:

  - decrease their activity level (burn fewer calories for the rest of the day)

  - satisfy their increased appetite through bigger portions and more frequent food consumption

  - reward themselves with high-calorie or unhealthy foods

- People tend to overestimate the amount of calories they've expended in a workout. As a result, they overcompensate with their eating behavior afterward.

- Excessive exercise may actually contribute to a deterioration of health. The body secretes the stress hormone cortisol with fatigue and muscle/joint aches. Cortisol causes fat to be deposited around the midsection of the body and can lead to metabolic syndrome.

- Low-intensity exercise, like walking, yoga, Pilates, hiking, and recreational biking and swimming, does not trigger the compensatory effects that are seen with stressful exercise.

- What we should have learned from Dr. Jean Mayer's studies in the 1960s is that the Energizer Bunny is always thinner than the Hulk.

- The health benefits of physical activity are tremendous when done *correctly*. Exercise helps to...

- improve psychological well-being/ boost mood
- reduce stress
- enhance mental clarity and acuity
- speed up metabolism
- support strong immune system functioning
- improve skin/complexion
- regulate the digestive system
- build stamina and strengthen the heart
- enhance work, recreation, and sport performance
- strengthen and maintain healthy muscles, bones, and joints
- reduce the risk of premature death and the development of numerous diseases

- Sustained energetic and productive movement throughout the day is best for weight management. Be one of the movers and shakers of the world.

~ 7 ~

The Skinny on How to Stay Lean

What Is the Optimal Balance of Food Groups?

Now *that* is a very controversial question. For over a century, people have been arguing about this very topic. Many nutritionists recommend the balance that is prescribed by the USDA—one that is best exemplified by either the MyPlate diet or the revamped food pyramid. I don't quite agree with this balance, no matter what geometrical shape it's put into. However, for the sake of fairness, we're going to hear their side of the story before we come to any conclusions.

The government didn't dabble in food advice until 1916, when we were smack-dab in the middle of World War I. With all the wartime rations and scarcities, the American government wanted to make sure that kids were getting enough food and taking in all the nutrients they needed for growth and health. At first, their recommendations were very nonspecific. But over time, the government decided to become more actively involved in establishing guidelines. By 1943, we were in the middle of another war—World War II. The government had cause to become concerned about nutrition once again, so they decided to make more precise dietary guidelines. That's when the "Basic Seven" came into fashion. Take a look at the USDA's 1943 idea of health.[1]

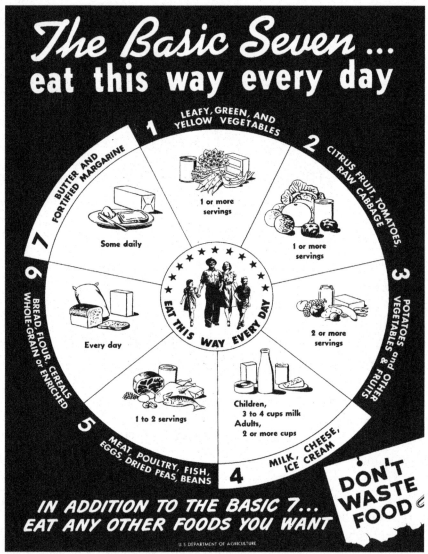

US Department of Agriculture

Don't you just love the fact that there's an entire category devoted to butter? Hahaha. I do! And the drawings and slogans are priceless.

Eventually, critics of the plan decided that these seven groups were too complex for most people. When 1956 rolled around, the list was shortened and streamlined. Thus, the "Basic Four" was born. It consisted of the following:[2]

1. four or more servings of bread/cereal (whole grain, enriched, or restored)
2. two or more servings of meat or alternatively dried beans, peas, or nuts
3. four or more servings of fruits/vegetables
4. milk

This categorization lasted for decades. The children of the sixties, seventies, and eighties grew up with it. But they never stopped growing up—and *out*. All of a sudden, no one needed to worry about the original problem—whether children were getting enough food. They were obviously getting too much. Something had gone terribly wrong, and it was time for another intervention.

In 1992, the original food pyramid was born. (If you need a recap of what it looks like, flip back to the "Introduction: A Disordered Eating Society.")[3] Unlike the Basic Seven and the Basic Four, the food pyramid's shape was able to depict the USDA's recommendations for portion sizes. The puny peak consisted of sugar/fat products. Consequently, devotees of this plan ate these foods sparingly. The big base consisted of carbohydrates like white flour, pasta, cereal, corn, and rice (foods that were considered nutritious and cheap). Accordingly, pyramid aficionados ate between six and eleven grain/carb servings per day. That's *not* counting all the carbohydrate servings they got through milk products, fruits, vegetables, and sweets. All in all, carbohydrate intake was excessive, to say the least. But no big deal. As long as those terrible, nasty, fattening fats were minimized, we were safe. Right?

What do you think happened? Did we slim down?

Negative. To everyone's great surprise, food pyramid enthusiasts took on the geometric shape of their diet plan.

By 2005, the food pyramid was revised. But the bottom tier of this version is whole-grain foods and plant oils. Still not right. So finally, in 2011, that food pyramid was thrown out too. The newest USDA fad is the MyPlate plan, which is supposed to provide the best illustration of portion sizes.[4]

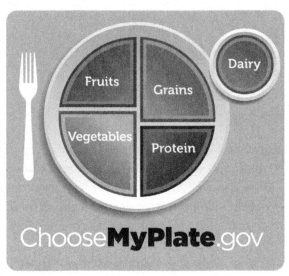

US Department of Agriculture

Pretty, isn't it? Too bad not much has changed. Take a look and see for yourself. Carbohydrates still make up more than three-fourths of the plate. There's no mention of fats at all. Sometimes, if you're lucky, you'll find a Mickey-Mouse-like version with a "fats" bubble on the upper left. But even then, the fats they typically recommend (salad dressing, nuts, peanut butter) are providing more carbohydrate calories, as well. And of course, the dairy bubble, which is most likely to be low-fat milk or yogurt, is an additional carb.

Do you see what they did? It's kind of like a magic trick, actually. They just rearranged the groupings! True, the portion size of grains has been somewhat diminished. But the overall composition is similar to that of the pyramid. The balance is still heavily weighted in favor of carbohydrates. And once again, fats and proteins are minimized.

So what is your prediction? Will the outcome of the MyPlate diet be any different from the food pyramid?

You don't need to be a rocket scientist to figure this one out.

Circle-shaped diet plans are no better than triangle-shaped diet plans when it comes to nutrition. If we really want to eliminate our society's nutritional problems, we absolutely must recognize that grains, starchy carbohydrates, sugars, and low fat, sweetened dairy products need to be minimized. In their stead, low-GI carbs (especially vegetables), proteins, and healthy fats need to be maximized.

In what proportions, though? How do we know the ideal ratio of carb:protein:fat to have in a day, or for that matter, in each meal?

Let's look at studies that examine diets with different proportions of each of these food groups and see which ones worked best. Though there are countless studies with this goal, I chose three so as not to bore you. Please stick with me as we consider this extremely important topic.

1. Our first study comes from the City of Hope Medical Center in Duarte, California.[5] Two groups of men were put on different diets; *they both had the same number of calories*, but one was low in fat and the other was higher in fat. After six months, the men on the high-fat diet lost 63 percent more weight than the men on the low-fat plan! Did you get that? The men who ate *more fat* and *less carbs* in their diet lost more weight.

2. The *New England Journal of Medicine* provided another great study on this matter.[6] Severely obese subjects were placed on either a low-carb diet or a high-carb/low-fat diet. Six months later, the low-carb dieters showed the greatest improvements in health. They lost more weight, had fewer side effects from insulin secretion, and had better lipid profiles (less fat in their blood)! That's rather mind-boggling. Eating a *low-fat* diet actually led to *more fat* in the blood in this study.

3. Perhaps the most compelling of all is the well-respected *A-to-Z* study published in the *Journal of the American Medical Association* in 2007.[7] This study compares four very different, leading diets. Here they are listed from the lowest carbohydrate intake to the highest:

    1. The Atkins Diet

        •   consists of protein, fats, and vegetable carbohydrates, no starchy carbs at all

    2. The Zone Diet

        •   uses a 40-30-30 ratio: 40 percent carbohydrates, 30 percent protein, 30 percent fat

3. The LEARN Diet

    • involves mostly carbohydrates, some protein, and very little fat

4. The Ornish Diet

    • consists almost completely of carbohydrates and a small amount of protein; fats are totally off-limits

Overweight women were placed on one of these four diets. The good news is over the next six months, they all steadily lost weight. Most important, the order of weight loss (from most to least) goes as follows:

Coming in first place—the Atkins Diet
Runner-up—The Zone Diet
Third Place—The LEARN Diet
And the loser is—The Ornish Diet

Did you catch the trend? The diets are in the same order as they were when I listed them from lowest carbohydrate intake to highest (a.k.a. highest protein/fat content to lowest). That means the people who achieved the *most rapid weight loss* were the ones eating the least amount of carbohydrates and the most protein and fat. But as you go down the list and the diets get higher in carbohydrates, the amount of weight loss decreases! If this had been a competition, the losers (not the weight losers), would be the Ornish dieters. They achieved the *least amount of weight loss*—because they ate almost all carbohydrates and very little protein and fat. After one year, the Atkins group had lost an average of ten pounds, while the Ornish dieters had lost only about four pounds.

Now, we should never measure overall health by the number on the scale. For this reason, the study also compared the women's blood pressure and lipid (blood-fat) test results. Here too, the no-meat, no-animal fat Ornish diet performed the worst, while the group that consumed the most animal products (the Atkins group) performed as well or better than all other groups. This surprises many who correlate high blood pressure and high lipid profiles with eating animal products. Granted, there are healthy and unhealthy types of this food group. It's not the McDonald's cheeseburgers and high-fat hot dogs that helped the Atkins dieters lose weight; rather, it's the wild-caught fish and grass-fed meat, the cheese and whole milk.

All the dieters from the study strayed from their prescribed diets throughout the year, as dieters almost always do. But guess which group found it easiest to stick to their diet. Guess which women were the most comfortable while losing weight. Again, it was the Atkins dieters. Since these women were not as calorie restricted, they didn't feel starved into weight loss.

Let me pause and make one important thing clear: I am not advocating a strict adherence to a diet like the Atkins diet, which eliminates carbohydrates completely. Going to any extreme is dangerous. Remember that I am a firm believer that *diets don't work* in general. However, I do believe that there are important lessons we can take away from these studies if we allow them to inform us about how our bodies react to various dietary imbalances.

Dissecting the Four Dietary Imbalances

high carb, *low fat*	high carb, *high fat*
low carb, *low fat*	low carb, *high fat*

We are now going to look at the consequences of each of these common nutritional imbalances, because they elicit very different states of health. As we do so, think about the people you know who have tried each one. Do any of them describe your diet?

High-Carb/Low-Fat Diet

High-car/low-fat is perhaps the most popular diet of the past few decades. It might yield some success in the short term, but in the long term, it's a downright failure. The only way to lose weight on this diet is to really restrict calories, to basically starve yourself. Since all carbs are easily converted to glucose, sugar intake is astronomical! Good, natural fats that are vital for satiation are removed from the diet, only to be replaced by carbohydrates and trans fats. That's the terrible twosome that is implicated in all sorts of disease processes! Essentially, people on this diet are *starving to obesity* (and all its related health issues).

High-Carb/High-Fat Diet

The all-American diet, this is for people who value taste over nutrition. After all, no one eats brownies, french fries, and cheesecake for their nutritional benefits. Very often, people on this diet believe all calories are equal. "If I have to restrict myself to only 1,500 calories per day, I might as well make those 1,500 calories as delicious as possible." Vegetarians and vegans can also fall into this category but for very different reasons. They need to get most of their protein through high-fat or high-carbohydrate protein sources, like peanut butter, tofu, and beans. Unfortunately, this diet simultaneously causes people to gain excess body fat and prevents them from burning existing fat off.

Low-Carb/Low-Fat Diet

Many programs use this diet to achieve *dramatic* weight loss. But remember, dramatic weight loss leads people into trouble (think: starvation periods that cause the metabolism to shut down and set people up for greater weight gain later). This diet does not skimp on protein, vitamins, fiber, or minerals, which is great! Still, it creates other nutritional deficiencies that stem from limited healthy fats and thus is not a diet I recommend.[8,9]

Low-Carb/High-Fat Diet

This is a good maintenance diet because it's easy to feel comfortable and satiated while receiving good nutrition. Fat storage is minimized. As long as the fats you eat are healthy fats and the carbohydrates you choose are nutrient-filled vegetables, you can steadily and safely lose weight on this plan.

Which of these four groups do you think the food pyramid diets and even the MyPlate diet fit into? I'd say the high-carb/low-fat category. Could this be why Americans are always fighting the battle of the bulge?

Here are my concluding remarks. Based on extensive research, my experience in practice, and the previously mentioned articles, I recommend that people eat plenty of protein and healthy fats and limit their carbohydrate intake. Most of your carb calories should stem from *stems*. Fill up on fiber-packed, water-filled, low-sugar vegetables like broccoli, leafy greens, and cauliflower. Of the starchier 20 percent carbohydrates (bananas, corn, grains, peas, beans, potatoes), choose only a few.

I'm not being very specific, I know. I am always wary of specifying numerical parameters for healthy eating because I want people to understand concepts rather than blindly follow rules. Adam and Eve didn't frolic around the Garden of Eden with a food scale. Neither should we conform our diets to an exact algorithm. Nevertheless, in order to give you an idea of what a healthy balance of food groups might look like, here's my suggestion:

35–45% low-GI carbs + 25–35% protein + 30–40% healthy fats
= 100% satisfaction.

Personally, I love this balance because it's satiating, nourishing, and safe—safe because it makes weight maintenance easy. Keep in mind, however, that these ranges represent percentages of total caloric intake, *not* volume. I'm not saying that 40 percent of your dinner plate should be loaded up with cheese and avocado. That would be way too much. As a matter of fact, that's one of my main qualms with the MyPlate diet; it does not illustrate portion sizes based on calories. Filling the grains triangle with compact, white, sticky rice would be very different than filling that same triangle with some popcorn.

The MyPlate diet visually proposes a diet of the following proportions: 75% carbs + 25% protein +/- a bit of fat. How radically different from what I am advocating! But don't forget, if we want dramatic improvement, we need dramatic change.

I'm sorry I'm not offering you a pretty rainbow-colored diagram. Worse still, the nebulous formula I presented requires you to do some work; you have to understand the calorie content and serving sizes of what you're eating. But the fact is, nutrition is complex, because your body is complex, beautifully complex.

Okay, now for the fun part of this chapter.

Once you understand the underlying concepts of what constitutes a healthy meal, you can get creative. For the rest of the chapter, we'll go through a variety of options for breakfast, lunch, dinner, and snacks that use the principles we've learned. But remember, all the meals I list here are just suggestions. Use that amazing imagination of yours to think up healthy meals that fit your own taste and lifestyle.

Ideas and Templates for Balanced, Satisfying, Diverse Meals

Breakfast

Option 1 (The Goldilocks): Start with hot oat bran cereal mixed with flaxseed meal. Add a glob of peanut or almond butter or maybe a dash of cinnamon, nutmeg, and/or cloves; a drop of vanilla or almond extract; nuts; fruit… If you find that you can't live without sweetness (but you keep giving it a shot!), add a tiny amount of a natural sweetener like honey, maple syrup, no-sugar-added natural fruit preserves, or agave nectar. I've even heard of people making oatmeal with milk, a sprinkle of Stevia, and fresh-squeezed lemon juice for a lemon-cream-pie effect. Pair this with some plain Greek yogurt or cottage cheese with strawberries.

Option 2 (I Do Not Like Green Eggs and Ham): Load a three-egg omelet with spinach, tomatoes, peppers, or any veggies you like. Sprinkle a little cheese in there if you'd like. Pair this with one piece of whole-grain, fibrous bread, toasted and spread with butter.

Option 3 (The Cereal Killer): Since cereals are typically highly refined and even the "healthy, whole grain" cereals are loaded with sugar and additives, you have to be especially careful to read ingredients lists/nutrition labels. If you're really craving cereal, try a small bowl of homemade or natural granola with whole fat or 2 percent milk. Couple this with two hard-boiled eggs for long lasting energy.

Option 4 (The Monster Mash): This is the breakfast that my daughter ate throughout her professional ballet career. Most people looked at her like she was crazy, but hey, it worked for her. A big bowl of plain Greek yogurt, berries or a cut-up fruit, two spoonfuls of oat bran, some flax seed meal, chia seeds, and a handful of nuts, all mixed into one big concoction.

Option 5 (Gift-Wrapped): A whole-wheat wrap with eggs, avocado, cheese, tomato, and salsa.

Option 6 (The European): A platter of thinly sliced deli meat, cheeses, cucumbers, tomatoes and olives, plus a slice of grainy bread and/or a whole fruit. For many Americans, this doesn't seem like breakfast food, but why not? Fresh ingredients are wonderful any time of the day.

Notes:

- Did you notice that each breakfast includes a rough carbohydrate, a protein source, and some fat? If not, check it out. That's key.

- It's especially important to hydrate in the morning. Tea or coffee is fine, but all of the day's meals and snacks are incomplete without a large glass of water.

- Avoid the PPPs (plaque-producing products): sweet rolls, sweet cereal, pancakes with syrup, and pastries.

- If you like to have the same breakfast almost every morning, fine! Personally, I choose to eat a bowl of Greek yogurt with one-third cup of blueberries and walnuts almost every morning.

- Remember that breakfast sets the tone for the day. Don't skip it! People who eat breakfast tend to be thinner than non–breakfast eaters. They also tend to be more active and energetic, and they make healthier food choices throughout the day. Non–breakfast eaters are liable to be more insulin reactive and more prone to fat storage.[10]

Lunch

Option 1 (The Wrapper): Chicken, cheese, avocado, and tomato rolled up in a whole-grain tortilla. Goes great with a whole fruit and some sugar snap peas to munch on.

Option 2 (Souper Salad): Couple a bowl of black bean soup with a chef salad. Include ham/turkey and hard-boiled eggs, plus flavor enhancers like cheese, bacon, mushrooms, avocado, and sunflower seeds. Lightly drizzle (rather than drench) olive oil and vinegar on top, letting the natural flavors of the salad come through.

Option 3 (The Popeye): A whole-grain sandwich loaded with meat, onions, lettuce, cheese and tomato, plus a side of cooked spinach.

Option 4 (In Your Face): Whole-grain crackers with deli meat and cheese piled on top—like mini-open-faced sandwiches. A side of carrots, a sliced-up cucumber/bell pepper, or an apple are perfect additions.

Option 5 (Homemade Gazpacho): Toss small slices of cucumber, chickpeas, fresh cilantro and/or parsley, diced peppers, tomatoes and/or onions, and small chunks of deli meat in a healthy oil, vinegar, salt, and pepper dressing. You can also crumble some cheese on top.

Option 6 (You Say Tomato, I Say Tomahto): A bowl of lentil soup and tuna salad in a scooped-out whole tomato.

Option 7 (Gourmet Chicken/Tuna Salad): If you really want to impress your friends, make your tuna or chicken salad with plain, whole-fat yogurt instead of mayo, some toasted (not candied) nuts, and celery slices. Play around with spices (curry? dill?).

Option 8 (Say "Cheese!"): Fold a whole-grain tortilla in half with Havarti cheese and spinach, and lightly fry in butter until melty. Add a chopped salad with romaine lettuce, asparagus, onions, tomatoes, and thinly sliced roast beef.

Snacks

Option 1 (Smooth Move): To make a fruit smoothie, put strawberries in a blender and add one cup of plain yogurt and shaved ice. (Play around with ingredients: peanut butter, flaxseed meal, chia seeds, half a banana, blueberries, whole milk, unsweetened cocoa powder, whey protein powder...) Blend and enjoy! This is how a healthy smoothie is done, unlike those sweetened, expensive ones at the mall. Smoothies are also a great breakfast option.

Option 2 (Hola Granola!): Make your own baggies of homemade granola. Mix low or no-sugar naked granola (or make it from scratch with any of the natural sweeteners I've mentioned) with almonds, pecans, or walnuts; coconut shavings; and a few raisins. Eat a small portion of this low-sugar granola on Greek yogurt.

Option 3 (Sweet and Salty): Celery with peanut butter. Easy peasy.

Option 4 (The Cheesehead): String cheese sticks and slices of red, yellow, orange, or green bell pepper.

Option 5 (Cottage in the Woods): Cottage cheese with chia seeds and berries or a plum.

Option 6 (The Jerk): Eat some beef or turkey jerky with raw veggies and/or fruit.

Option 7 (Cracked Up): Have whole grain crackers with cheese.

Option 8 (The Egghead): Make two hard-boiled eggs and eat with fruit and/or raw veggies.

Option 9 (The Body Builder): If you can find a high-fiber, high-protein bar that isn't saturated with artificial sweeteners, by all means, go for it. But do your research. A good bar will have as many or more grams of fiber than it does sugar, and not have a long list of scary-sounding ingredients.

*If you're still hungry, make sure that you're hydrated. Water, fruit, and veggies provide the bulk you need for satiation.

Dinner

Option 1 (Somethin's Fishy): Salmon, quinoa, broccoli, and arugula salad with lightly drizzled dressing.

*Pro tip: homemade dressing is surprisingly easy to make. Get creative with a healthy oil, flax seed meal for thickening, herbs/spices and perhaps vinegar, lemon juice or even buttermilk (for a creamy dressing). This ensures that your homemade salad dressing isn't like its manufactured counterparts, which are typically tantamount to a fattening chemical soup.

Option 2 (Holy Guacamole): Fish tacos made with corn or whole-wheat tortillas, white fish, guacamole/salsa, cilantro, and stir-fried bell peppers and onions. Add a big salad loaded with vegetables and sprinkled with sunflower seeds or veggies with guacamole dip.

Option 3 (Year-Round Thanksgiving): Start with turkey cutlets and then throw into the oven a variety of vegetables to roast until crunchy on the outside. Include a sweet potato (don't forget that potato skins contain much of the root's fiber and nutrients!), and dress it in butter and cinnamon for extra deliciousness.

Option 4 (My Thai): Shrimp and heaps of veggies (broccoli, peppers, spinach, mushrooms, onions, bok choy) stir-fried with sesame oil or coconut oil, ginger, and garlic over a half cup of brown rice. You can sprinkle peanuts and fresh cilantro on top, too.

Option 5 (Steak and Potatoes): Use lean, grass-fed steak. Steam cauliflower and white cabbage until soft and then mash them up with some butter. Okay, so there're no potatoes in the "Steak and Potatoes" dinner. But you better believe it: mashed cauliflower and cabbage is better tasting and better for you.

Option 6 (Rainy Day Special): Upgrade that feel-good meal of chicken soup by adding barley, leeks, onions, mushrooms, wilted spinach, carrots, and celery. Pair this with a salad that includes sliced avocado or blue/goat/parmesan/mozzarella cheese.

Option 7 (Pork Barrel): Pulled pork with brown rice and Cuban-spiced black beans. Get your greens with a serving of brussels sprouts and a salad.

Option 8 (The Italian Stallion): Whole-wheat spaghetti with lean ground meat or homemade meatballs, zucchini, sun-dried tomatoes, and mushrooms. Instead of tomato sauce (full of sugar) or Alfredo sauce (heavy with fat), use olive oil, Italian seasoning, and garlic. Finish it off with a salad. (Pasta is fine as long as it's in a small quantity and balanced with plenty of greens and meat).

Option 9 (Cheeseburger in Paradise): Make homemade burgers with lean ground, grass-fed beef, ground turkey, or ground grass-fed buffalo or bison meat. For a gourmet burger, mix chopped onions, garlic, peppers, and spices into the meat. You can add any kind of cheese you like on top. For the healthiest version, use a large lettuce leaf as your bun. Or put tomato, raw onion, lettuce, cheese, and mustard on top and then use a fork and knife to eat. A side of green beans with butter will complete this meal.

Option 10 (Healthy Taco Salad): Romaine lettuce leaves loaded with chicken, pork, beef, or fish; guacamole or avocado; salsa; shredded cheese; beans; sautéed peppers and onions; and fresh herbs. Don't put it in a taco shell, and there's no need to add rice. The beans are plenty of carbs for this meal!

Okay, okay, I'm done. But I could've kept going. You see, once you know the principles of healthy eating, the possibilities become endless! It's like math; if you know the formula, you can make the variables whatever you want and it will always be right. For meal planning, here's the only formula you need:

A variety of food groups with an emphasis on
fiber-rich vegetables and protein

+

Whole foods that have not been refined or adulterated

=

One very healthy meal

Summary
The Skinny on How to Stay Lean

- Since 1916, the government has promoted various nutritional recommendations in accordance with evolving political agendas as well as evolving scientific understanding.

- When four major diet plans were compared in terms of overall weight loss, sense of well-being, blood-lipid profile, and ease of adherence to the diet, the clear winner was the low-carb Atkins diet. The Ornish diet (high-carb, low-protein, low-fat) came in last place.

- The MyPlate diet looks more like the Ornish diet than the Atkins diet. Visually, it proposes a diet of the following proportions: 75 percent carbs + 25 percent protein +/- a bit of fat. With this estimation, the MyPlate diet has not strayed far from the original food pyramid.

- The best diet for *rapid weight loss* and for those with serious health issues is the low-carb, low-fat diet.

- The best diet for *weight maintenance* is the low-carb, high-healthy-fat, high-protein diet. It provides complete nutrition, satiety, and mood stability while minimizing fat storage.

- There is no precise formula for perfect health, but the range I suggest is as follows:

  - 35–45% low-GI carbs + 25–35% protein + 30–40% healthy fats

~ 8 ~

Miracle Foods or Poison?

Picture this: you are the owner of a brand-new Rolls Royce. Imagine its sleek design, the beautiful leather interior, and the powerful engine. As the proud owner of this exquisite piece of machinery, of course you want to take meticulous care of it. You would never, ever put crude oil into its gas tank. Well-made cars cannot perform optimally without a consistent supply of high-quality energy.

We are all worth infinitely more than the most expensive car ever made. But guess what. A lot of people treat their cars much better than they treat their own bodies.

Humans perform poorly with inadequate or inconsistent supplies of energy, just like their cars. When cheap, shoddy fuel is poured into our tanks, we suffer with mood problems, fatigue, sugar highs, sugar lows, frustrating brain fog, weight problems, and the invisible internal clogging of our transmission. No one is exempt. High-calorie, nutrient-poor sludge alters even the most vigorous and vivacious of adolescents, athletes, and seemingly healthy individuals. After all, youth and resiliency are not eternal. Eventually, the progressive internal damage that has been occurring for years behind the scenes becomes visible on the surface, too.

We need to determine which kinds of food are cheap crude oil and which are premium-grade fuel. Just like gasoline, the right kinds of fuel can help you function much better and run for much longer.

In this chapter, we will examine four of our society's main sources of fuel: corn, soy, vegetable oils, and sugar. Without these products, our current grocery stores would be depleted of food. They are the cornerstone of our diets and our agricultural economy. Since corn, soy, vegetable oils, and sugar are in most of what we eat, we have to understand how they affect our bodies and our environment.

Have you ever heard the saying, "You are what you eat?" However silly this expression may seem, there is some physiologic truth to it. Based on this concept, we are …

Corn

Yup, we are all walking corn husks. We and the livestock that we consume have become corn by-products.

Let's use the chicken nuggets that we grew up on as an example. First of all, the chicken is corn-fed. Then, cornstarch is laced into the meat mixture to glue it together. And of course, corn forms some of the batter surrounding the chicken. Next, the cook takes the corn/chicken conglomerate and fries it in—you guessed it—corn oil. By this time, the consumer is probably craving some much-needed corn to make up for the lack of corn in their corn feast. So it's all washed down with some type of corn-syrup-sweetened beverage.

We're eating corn all the time without even realizing it, because it's often disguised under one of the following aliases: dextrin, malto-dextrin, dextrose, glucose, fructose, high fructose, corn sugar, lecithin, sorbitol, vegetable starch, vegetable oil, maize, thickeners, sweeteners, and syrup.

Is this really a bad thing though? After all, we also have corn to thank for countless culinary delights, like barbecue sauce, mustard, ketchup, mayo, salad dressings, marbled beef, soft drinks, cereal, coffee creamers, candy, jelly, Jell-O, gravies, sauces, chewing gum, and chips, not to mention the more obvious—corn on the cob, creamed corn, cornbread, grits, popcorn, kettle corn, corn dogs … Corn makes everything so much better, doesn't it?

To answer this question, I'm going to do my best to highlight some of the brilliant work of Michael Pollan. In his two fabulous books, *The Omnivore's Dilemma* and *In Defense of Food*, he exposes the connections between our overconsumption of refined carbohydrates and our societal obesity epidemic.[1, 2]

Most of the eighty million acres of corn produced in the United States becomes the main ingredient in livestock feed, which enables the *rapid fattening* of cows, chickens, and even farm-raised fish.[3] The heavy starch from the corn makes animal muscles become striated with fat, called *marbling*. And that's exactly why Americans love corn-fed meat; when all the muscles are lined with fat, it becomes terribly juicy.

Grass-fed beef, on the other hand, is not nicely marbled. In fact, it's lean. It has a different taste than corn-fed beef because it has a different composition of fats; specifically, it's rich in omega-3 fatty acids. Do you remember omega-3's from "How Our Bodies Use Food"? If not, think the kings of nutrition, which boost brain function and reduce inflammation and the risk of cancer, heart disease, and psychiatric disorders.

That miracle-worker fat is not found in corn-fed beef like it is in grass-fed. Yet farmers will choose to feed their livestock corn-based products nine times out of ten. Why? It's obviously not for health reasons.

No, the reason is money, of course. Economics drives agricultural practices. Raising livestock in crowded feedlots or fish in ponds, feeding them with inexpensive corn, and then watching them quickly fatten up leads to a larger profit margin. I'll give you one guess as to what they invest their profits in.

Yup, it's corn.

I said that there's a physiologic truth to the saying "You are what you eat ..." Well, when it comes to our meat, we grow to reflect the marbled-fat composition of our livestock. If Sweeney Todd and Miss Lovett were to fillet an American, they'd probably be happy to find juicy fat striated throughout the musculature, just like our meat sources, thanks to our corn-based and corn-fed diet.

Sadly, you'll have to be prepared to pay an arm and a leg for wild-caught fish, wild game, and grass-fed beef. Eating food the way God intended it to be isn't cheap. That's why even knowledgeable Americans choose to save a little money at the grocery store instead of grabbing the healthier option. But this penny-wise, pound-foolish philosophy contributes to our growing problems with diabetes, obesity, and cardiovascular disease. So in our efforts to save money, we pay a far higher price—our future health.

The story doesn't end there, for we haven't even touched on the tragic consequences that our corn-fed meat industry has on the animals it profits from.

Look at the feedlot cow. She is guaranteed a short life, one in which she can hardly move about because of overcrowding. She suffers with constant eye irritation thanks to the manure dust blowing everywhere. But worst of all, she suffers from the chronic pain and sickness that comes with a feedlot diet.

Cows can't be thrown onto this corn diet all at once. They have to be transitioned into it over time with increasing amounts of formula until they are adequately adjusted. What's in the unnatural formula they're force-fed? Well, corn is the number-one ingredient, of course. Liquefied fat, protein supplements, liquid vitamins, synthetic estrogen, antibiotics, alfalfa, and silage (fermented crops) make up the rest of this mixture.

Instinctively, animals wouldn't consume their own species. Yet the "liquefied fat" in this formula is beef fat. We've managed to get them to do something abhorrent to their intuition. By disguising their fat with the feedlot mixture, we've taken away their ability to naturally reject cannibalism. A hundred years ago, cattle were also fed beef protein remnants. When we found a connection between the cattle that consumed beef protein and mad cow disease, the practice was abandoned. Finally, the FDA officially put a stop to the practice of forced protein cannibalism. But forced fat cannibalism still abounds.

What does this diet do to the naturally herbivorous cows? Since they are given massive doses of carbohydrates and they don't get to exercise, they mature very quickly, which is exactly what the cattle farmers want. Thus, fat accounts for a large percentage of their body weight, including that which adulterates their muscle tissue.

Worse yet, the feedlot formula causes livestock terrible bloating and gas—a gas unlike anything human beings have experienced. The pressure from this terrible gas squeezes the cow's lungs, even to the point of suffocation. *Bloat*, or *acidosis*, is the name of the resulting condition, the consequence of a diet high in starch and low in fiber. Once they develop acidosis, cows stop eating and suffer from diarrhea, liver disease, and a weakened immune system. They become more susceptible to every bacterial and viral illness imaginable, making infection extremely prevalent. Furthermore, the cows' crowded living conditions worsen the complications stemming from infection. That's why cows have to be put on so many antibiotics.

The overuse of antibiotics in cattle is one of the biggest contributing factors to a serious problem in our society: drug-resistant bacteria.

In other words, bacteria that cause infections we can't treat with modern medicine.

With this life of chronic pain, sickness, and heinous treatment, it's no surprise that cows can't last much longer than 150 days—the amount of time it takes to get them fat enough for slaughter. They just get too sick. They end up dying from one of the ailments mentioned above. I'm not a touchy-feely, cuddle-up-to-a-cow kind of person. Still, this type of animal cruelty makes my blood boil.

As if it weren't enough that our corn-fed culture is ruining the health of both humans and livestock alike, it's also harming our environment. On sunny days, if you take a walk through the fields of our heartland and trail behind a harvesting tractor, you'll find some really big footprints. Carbon footprints. Fifty gallons of oil per acre of corn is consumed through transportation, the production of chemicals, and the use of tractors, drying equipment, and harvesting equipment! Forget about the old days of reaping free food from God's green earth, using only sunshine and natural nutrients found in soil. For every calorie of corn produced, one calorie of fossil fuels is expended. And unless the price of fossil fuels rises, this extravagant waste is here to stay.

In the past, farmers could not raise corn year after year; they had to rotate crops. Corn zaps too much nitrogen from the soil. But thanks to modern technology, we've found a way to bypass nature yet again. With the advent of ammonium nitrate (a substance developed for making explosives) and pesticides (a substance developed as poison gas for war), there's no need to rotate crops. Now farmers can produce corn year after year with even greater yields. Where in the 1920s, one acre of land produced about twenty bushels of corn, it now can produce about two hundred! Isn't it amazing what these poisons can do for us?

Of course, everything comes at a price. Those nitrogen fertilizers and pesticides that saturate our farm soil don't just vanish. They flow into our streams and rivers, polluting everything in their course. They affect the flora and fauna of every area they touch, shrinking the biodiversity of species. Ultimately, the poisons terminate in the Gulf of Mexico. This leads to an overgrowth of algae, which in turn leads to large, hypoxic dead zones that are incapable of supporting normal marine life.

Do you know how valuable manure fertilizer was for farmers in past decades? As a little girl, I recall needing to plug my nose whenever we drove through farmland. Sometimes, the dramatic child in me would think that I could just die from the horrid smell of manure everywhere. Once, I remember my dad looking at me as we drove, rolling down the window, and saying with a smile, "Mmmm, money."

What? I thought. *You are so weird!* Soon after, I learned that he wasn't relishing the rotten-egg smell; he was appreciating the fact that manure was the elixir of life for soil. He knew that it turned average dirt into rich, fertile ground. But that's only true about manure from natural, healthy cows.

Today, many farmers won't even use manure that comes from feed-lot cows. Why? Because the waste's nitrogen and phosphorus levels are too high. It ruins their crops. No longer is their manure the liquid gold that generates life. Instead, it is the toxic waste that kills organisms as it dissipates into rivers and streams.[4, 5]

If the very waste that comes from corn-fed cows is so incredibly toxic, imagine how toxic the poor cows' bodies are. What do you think?

- If the cows' by-products are too poisonous for crops, why are they okay for us? Exactly what toxins are we ingesting when we sink our teeth into a burger or steak?

- What added hormones are we ingesting? Could this have something to do with our society's epidemic of hormonal imbalances? Since weight issues and hormones go hand in hand, could this even have something to do with the obesity epidemic?

- And what are all the negative consequences of adding antibiotics to feed mixture? Could that be creating an army of antibiotic-resistant bacteria?

I don't know ... Do some research. You may be the future in food science. Maybe I'll be buying *your* book soon.

The story of corn needed to be told. I want you to use your wisdom about the evolution of food products to see through all of the marketing madness. I want you to see how the greed in agribusiness has driven our patterns of food consumption. We are too often fed the wrong substances for the wrong reasons, to satiate the wrong people.

The incentive for food purchase in future generations must be health. So it all starts with you. Your buying power during upcoming decades will determine agricultural practices. If you dislike the demolition of your health, the animal cruelty, and the environmental destruction taking place due to modern agricultural practices, choose to boycott products made with corn syrup, choose to eat grass-fed meats, choose to limit your intake of unnatural products.

On that note, we must cover another plant that has corrupted our consumption practices and undermined our health.

Soy

Along with corn, soy deserves special coverage in this book. Thanks to Kaayla T. Daniel, PhD, CCN, we finally know the truth about soy, as the title of her book, *The Whole Soy Story: The Dark Side of America's Favorite Health Food*, promises.[6] And what a story it is!

Soy, the small legume *that comprises about 78 percent of the typical American's total fat intake*, is heralded as a miracle food—the supposed cure for cancer and menopause, a means of lowering high cholesterol levels, the nonallergenic dairy substitute, and a cheap protein to feed the masses. In essence, it is the answer to a vegan's quest for the holy grail of vegetable products. But even if you're not vegan or vegetarian, soy comprises a large part of your diet. Just like corn, it's a master of disguise, hidden in countless products with aliases like MSG, vegetable-protein isolates, SPI, soy protein isolate, textured vegetable protein, textured plant protein, TVP, lecithin, vegetable oil, vegetable broth, bouillon, natural flavor, and monodiglyceride.

With those pseudonyms, soy is used to jack up the protein content of everything from ravioli to hamburgers, shakes, chicken nuggets, and protein bars. Its by-products are incorporated into bread, ice cream, cake mixes, lemonade mixes, doughnuts, and numerous other packaged items. Moreover, soy fats are the chief fat used for cooking fast food and fried foods, they make up most margarines, and they are the primary ingredient in vegetable oil.

And what about all the times we consciously choose to eat soy, too? Think soy milk, soy sauce, toasted soy nuts, tofu and all tofu-based concoctions, soy flour, soy protein powder, soy chips, miso soup, edamame (soy beans) …

Wow. How did we fall so in love with soy?

Let's go back to the beginning, to the birth of this miracle food / toxin.

Contrary to popular belief, soy was not historically the ancient Asian food staple. In fact, its evolution to becoming an edible product is relatively recent. Around 200 BC, soy was first used by Asian cultures as a cover crop, or rather, *green manure*. Once farmers discovered that it enriches soil by fixing nitrogen into the earth, they used soybean plants in their crop rotation so that they could grow other valuable produce.

At that time, the Chinese considered the soybean inedible. They understood that it was toxic, even after ordinary cooking. Eventually, they figured out how to make soy digestible: fermentation.

Fast-forward many centuries to the 1930s, when soy found its major American sponsors. It was John Kellogg and Henry Ford who put this bean on its seemingly unstoppable course toward success. Both John Kellogg (of Kellogg cereal) and Henry Ford (founder of Ford Motor Company) found the soybean fascinating. They continuously searched for innovative uses for soy. In Europe, during the same time period, Hitler was extolling the virtues of a healthy, vegetarian lifestyle and promoting the consumption of soy.

The practical uses for soy seemed endless. Some people claimed that soy increased mental vitality and physical stamina. Henry Ford loved the bean and proposed using it in plastic products, cars, clothing, and refrigerators. The Soviets pushed for soy to be the low-cost solution to feed the masses. Castro encouraged massive soy production to nourish his country, as well. In fact, his perspective on soy became a beacon of light for other developing countries.

Starting in the 1980s, taxpayers unknowingly contributed to the funding of the NIH studies that would *prove* soy's health benefits. Results were inconclusive at best. Scientists hired by soy companies provided sketchy studies that claimed soy could tackle heart disease, cancer, menopause, and osteoporosis.

Advertisers purposely targeted the upper class, thinking that if they could get rich people to pay high prices for this miraculous "health food," then everyone else would follow suit.

> Just imagine you could grow the perfect food. This
> food not only would provide affordable nutrition, but

also would be delicious and easy to prepare in a variety of ways. It would be a healthful food, with no saturated fat. In fact, you would be growing a virtual fountain of youth on your back forty. This ideal food would help prevent, and perhaps reverse, some of the world's most dreaded diseases. You could grow this miracle crop in a variety of soils and climates. Its cultivation would build up, not deplete, the land ... this miracle food already exists ... It's called soy.[7] (Dean Houghton in John Deere's *The Furrow* magazine)

Today, the marketing push continues as soybean producers are obligated to give a percentage of their net profits to the United Soybean Board (USB). About eighty million dollars is collected annually to promote and strengthen soy's position in global markets.

Why is this a problem? After all, every mass-produced product, food or otherwise, has to have sponsors and marketing initiatives.

Here is a fun fact pulled directly from the book *The Whole Soy Story*. "While the Food and Drug Administration (FDA) has approved a heart health claim for soy protein, the agency also lists soy in its 'Poisonous Plant Database.' A search of the word soy in the database reveals 256 references, including studies that warn about goiters, growth problems, amino acid deficiencies, mineral malabsorption, endocrine disruption and carcinogenesis."[8]

The FDA is associating these horrific health problems with soy, and yet we are still hearing that it's a superfood. Something isn't adding up.

How is soy actually used by our bodies?

Soy products contain several chemicals that cause harm to our bodies, many of which are released because of the way it's processed. The soybean is actually one of the most processed foods out there, undergoing heavy-duty scrubbing and grinding, heat, alkali treatments, soaking, and refining before it's runway ready. Eventually, every bit of the soybean is used—toxins and all. Not bad for a product that started out as refuse!

Soy contains enzyme inhibitors that block our body's enzymatic digestion of protein. Do you see the tremendous irony there? *People eat soy for its protein content, yet they are ingesting a substance that actually undermines protein digestibility.* Soy literally depletes nutrients from your body.

The trypsin inhibitor (antinutrient) is actually deactivated in the process of fermentation, which validates the ancient Chinese wisdom that soy is inedible unless fermented. Yet sadly, in the shortened, efficient fermentation process we've invented, the enzyme inhibitor is not deactivated. Thus, the antinutrient remains in the soy we consume. No wonder soy often causes gastric upset (gas), decreased protein digestion, and chronic amino acid (protein) deficiencies.

Do you remember how we talked about phytates in "How Our Bodies Use Food"? Phytates block our body's ability to take up essential minerals like calcium, zinc, iron, and magnesium, all of which are essential for brain, body, and immune function. While all beans contain phytates, soy has the highest content of all legumes. These phytates are also not adequately removed through cooking.

Hemagglutinin—another substance in soy that should terrify us— is a clot-forming substance that causes red blood cells to clump together. Not the best thing for heart health, to say the least. Hemagglutinins are also growth-retarding substances, as are the trypsin inhibitors I mentioned earlier.

We haven't even finished yet. Many hormonal problems are related to the ingestion of soy products. The isoflavones in soybeans mimic the female hormone estrogen. Menopausal women and celibate monks might revel in the estrogen-like qualities of soy's isoflavones, but for the rest of the population, soy's hormonal qualities are detrimental, even dangerous. Men who regularly ingest soy reportedly have a lower sex drive and suffer from infertility problems. Children can experience a premature onset of puberty.

Most detrimental of all are soy's effects on infants. Soy has six hundred times the amount of estrogen-type compounds that a baby requires, or the equivalent of about five birth control pills per day—for a baby! Furthermore, soy milk has two hundred times the amount of manganese found in breast milk. Deficiency syndromes, hormonal problems, and growth problems have been linked to our misguided use of soy in baby formula, and we're still learning about all the behavioral, motor, and mental consequences. And to think that one-fourth of bottle-fed babies are given soy milk!

SPI, or soy protein isolate, is used in protein bars, protein powders, and anything in which a company profits by boosting protein content. Since I am a huge proponent for eating more protein, this should be a red flag to you: stay away from this kind of protein. Let's look at how soy protein isolate is manufactured.

First, soybeans are mixed with an *alkali solution to remove the fiber.* Once the fiber has been removed, an *acid wash in aluminum* tanks separates the product. While in these tanks, the soy picks up and holds on to high levels of aluminum. The precipitate from the acid wash is once again *neutralized in an alkaline solution.* Nitrates (which are cancer-producing) and a toxin called lysinoanlanine are formed during this alkaline processing. The resulting toxic, aluminum-filled curds are then *spray-dried at high temperatures* to achieve a fine, dry powder. Finally, *numerous additional chemical flavorings* (like MSG) are added to the mixture to minimize the nasty gunpowder taste and to infuse the final product with flavor.

I don't know what to call it, but that's not food anymore. Nothing about that process is natural.

Before I exhaust the topic of soy, I must address some of the environmental concerns associated with soy production.

Monsanto, the largest global soy-producing company, has engineered a genetically modified strain of soy that is resistant to a particular herbicide. Unfortunately for them, their plan backfired; some of the weeds that they were trying to kill became resistant to the herbicide as well. When the herbicide glyphosate was sprayed over an entire soybean farm, these superweeds did not die, but the bacteria that allow them to rot did. So the farms became filled with soybean plants that were covered in poison along with superweeds that were lying dormant, unable to decay. Not surprisingly, this situation has produced terrible outcomes. People living in these toxic areas have suffered with all sorts of illnesses. Farmers reported the death of livestock along with numerous cases of birth defects in newborn animals. In Argentina, for example, farms that once grew lentils, vegetables, and fruits have been transformed into acres of chemical wasteland.

These tragic circumstances beg some important questions. When we eat soy, how much of this poisonous herbicide are we ingesting? And if the herbicide kills bacteria in the soil, what is it doing to our bodies and the healthy bacteria that keep us running?

Soybean crops have replaced many indigenous crops in countries around the globe, which causes small farm owners to go out of business and leads to the loss of biodiversity in agriculture. Keep in mind that the repeated consumption of the same strain of any crop (due to the loss of agricultural biodiversity) seems to be increasing the frequency of food allergies in our society.

Personally, I think I've learned enough about this toxic product to minimize my intake of tofu and soy sauce. But you don't have to take my word for it; please, research this issue in greater depth through the Internet or by reading *The Whole Soy Story* and make up your own mind.

Let's move on to the next source of fuel I'd like us to examine: vegetable oils. We touched on them a bit in "How Our Bodies Use Food" when we looked at our unhealthily high consumption of omega-6 fats. Well, I'm afraid that we have to return to the discussion, because unfortunately, there's a lot more bad news when it comes to this food source.

Vegetable Oils

In her article, "The Dangers of Polyunsaturated Vegetable Oils," Sally Fallon reports,

> In test animals, diets high in ***polyunsaturates from vegetable oils*** inhibit the ability to learn, especially under conditions of stress; are toxic to the liver; compromise the integrity of the immune system; depress the mental and physical growth of infants; increase levels of uric acid in the blood; cause abnormal fatty acid profiles in the adipose tissues: have been linked to mental decline and chromosomal damage and accelerate aging.[9]

Please reread that slowly and let it sink in. This is what it says about the supposedly "heart-healthy" oils?

Vegetable oil and its offshoots: canola, palm, sunflower, safflower, cottonseed, grapeseed, peanut oil, and two from the topics we discussed above—corn and soybean oil—are some of the most highly processed, unnatural, and unhealthy products out there. That goes for the solidified forms, as well: margarine and other fake butter products.

Take a minute to study this graphical representation of the fabrication of these products and see for yourself:

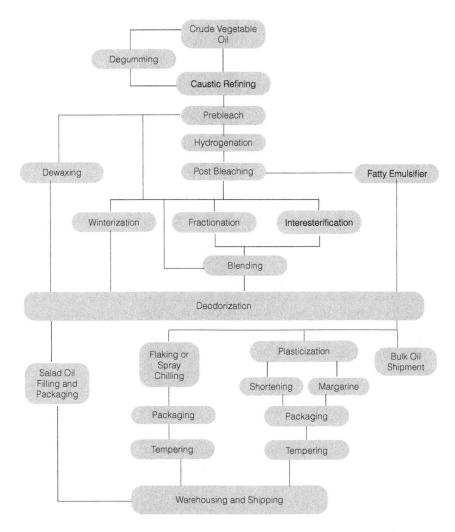

I don't know about you, but anytime words like *caustic refining*, *deodorizing*, *prebleaching* and *postbleaching*, and *plasticization* are used to describe the cooking of my food, I'd rather not put that so-called "food" in my body.

Compare this process to butter-making.

Step 1: Milk cow.
Step 2: Let cream separate naturally.
Step 3: Skim off cream.
Step 4: Shake until it becomes butter.[10]

During the manufacturing process, many chemicals are added to vegetable oil products, including butylated hydroxyanisole (BHA) and butylated hydroxytoluene (BHT). These two toxic substances have been found to be correlated with reproductive problems, high cholesterol, immune system damage, and liver and kidney problems. More harmful chemicals and pesticides than just these two are incorporated into vegetable oil production.

Canola oil, the star player in this team of oils, is a modified version of rapeseed oil. Rapeseed oil comes from the cotton plant—yes, the same cotton that makes up our clothes—and has a high level of poisonous erucic acid. In order to remove this poison from the soon-to-be canola oil, petroleum solvent is used under very high temperatures. After more acid, heat, and chemical treatments, the result is finally palatable. Called low erucic acid rapeseed (LEAR), this chemical soup was christened canola oil in 1980 as a marketing ploy.[11]

In "How Our Bodies Use Food," we discussed how our society eats about twenty times the amount of omega-6's as it should, which puts us at risk for cancer, heart disease, obesity, and diabetes, to name a few. We also examined how omega-6's are easily oxidized with light or heat exposure—whether on a grocery store shelf, during cooking, or in our bodies. And this oxidization depletes our bodies of *antioxidants*, which causes numerous deficiencies along with inflammation and cell mutation, the beginnings of many disease states. I remind you of this information because, as you recall, vegetable oils are high in omega-6 fatty acids.

In an article entitled, "Margarine Intake and Subsequent Coronary Heart Disease in Men," the authors chronicled a study of two groups of men, differentiated by their consumption of either butter or margarine.[12] After two decades of research, the results were stunning: During the second decade, the incidence of heart disease in the margarine group was 77 percent higher than that of the butter group!

Wow. The fascinating part to me is when you look at graphs of the rise of heart disease, diabetes, and obesity over the past century, they seem to be correlated with the rise of vegetable oil use. We can't, of course, say that the first trend is caused by the latter, but it does make you think. Could any of this be why, for the first time in modern history, children are expected to have a shorter life span than their parents?

As you ponder this question, we'll end with one final quote by Fallon, from the article mentioned earlier:

> What the scientific literature does tell us is that *low fat diets* for children, or diets in which *vegetable oils have been substituted for animal fats*, result in failure to thrive—failure to grow tall and strong—as well as learning disabilities, susceptibility to infection and behavioral problems. Teenage girls who adhere to such a diet risk reproductive problems. If they do manage to conceive, their chances of giving birth to a low birth weight baby, or a baby with birth defects, are high.[13]

This is obviously a type of food that we want to avoid. Unfortunately vegetable oils, like corn and soy, are everywhere in almost every packaged, manufactured, or fried food out there. Still, I'm willing to do whatever it takes to prevent the barrage of health problems these foods supply. What about you?

Sugar

Permit me to start with a trivia question. If you were stranded on a desert island, do you think you'd survive longer on sugar-water or just water?

Hold on to your answer, and I will tell you a tale of sailors who, in 1793, found themselves marooned on an island for nine days. Can you guess what their shipwrecked vessel was carrying? Sugar. Well, they had rum too—so more sugar in other words.

Only five sailors survived the nine days; their bodies were wasted away. The truth is, while water alone can keep a person alive for up to two weeks, sugar and water can kill you. How is this possible? How is it that something we consider *food* has the power to hasten our death?

I'll keep my explanation short and *sweet*.

Refined sugar, or sucrose, is different than glucose, which the body produces; fructose, which comes from fruit; and lactose, the sugar in dairy products. This type of sugar is man-made, created through a so-called *purifying* process that strips sugar cane and beets of all nutrients, including any vitamins, minerals, and fiber. The words *purified* and *refined* make it sound like this manufactured product is somehow purged of all its imperfections—polished, perfected, improved upon. What excellent word manipulation! In truth, the purification process leaves nothing but empty, naked calories with no nutritional value.

Even those words are misleading, however. Refined sugar is worse than emptiness or nakedness; it is actively destructive. It makes the body more acidic, and in an effort to recalibrate, the body releases minerals into the bloodstream. That's why sugar ingestion depletes the body of minerals like sodium, potassium, magnesium, and calcium. A diet consistently high in refined sugar causes so much calcium depletion that teeth and bones start to decay and weaken.

Have you ever pondered what humans did before Oral-B toothbrushes and Crest toothpaste came to save us from the horrors of tooth decay? Well, here's your answer: they didn't eat refined foods. As Harvard professor Ernest Hooten wrote in his book *Apes, Men and Morons*, "Let us cease pretending that toothbrushes and toothpaste are any more important than shoe brushes and shoe polish. It is store food that has given us store teeth."[14]

Alas, tooth and bone decay are not even the half of it. If a high-sugar diet persists, the liver, which stores excess sugar, balloons up. Eventually, it decides enough is enough and begins to send the sugar-turned-glycogen to the most unused parts of the body (i.e., the belly, butt, and breasts). When the sugar consumption continues (as it probably will since sucrose is an addictive substance), fat starts to build in and around vital organs, like the heart and kidneys. Over time, all organs are affected; their tissue degenerates, and they lose the ability to function.

I could continue to explain the possible consequences of incessant sugar ingestion (including brain damage and cellular death), but I promised to be succinct. So I'll wrap up with an interesting observation by Dr. William Coda Martin. In 1957, he set out to define what makes an edible substance poisonous. The definition he landed on was, "Any substance applied to the body, ingested or developed within the body which causes or may cause disease."[15] Considering what you've read about sucrose, are you surprised that Dr. Martin classified sugar as a poison?

Finding the Silver Lining

This was a heavy chapter, and I apologize for being the bearer of bad news. The bright side is that there are ways to circumvent the toxicity of the all-American diet. Here are some tips:

- Only buy and eat food that looks like real food, not synthetic imitations. Grocery stores set up their products in a way that makes this easy and convenient. The perimeter of the store is filled with real, nutritious, naturally edible foods (vegetables, fruit, meat, dairy) while the middle aisles are filled with un-natural, processed foods. Stay on the periphery, and you'll be good to go.

- Here's another tip: avoid purchasing boxes filled with mysterious ingredients and packaged so the food will never rot. That's not normal. Food rots! If you can't pronounce the ingredients on the back of the packaging, then put that puppy back on the shelf. The more ingredients, the more synthetic and processed a product is likely to be. Stick with food that is natural and preservative-free.

- Consider buying organic and local grown. It's worth the extra cost if you think about the medical bills you're saving on later.

- Make sure to wash produce off thoroughly. I used to swipe my apples and berries under the faucet carelessly, thinking that I was just trying to wash away dirt and a little dirt never hurt anyone. But actually, it's more critical than that; a scrupulous washing helps remove harmful pesticides and chemicals.

Finally, consider what your food source was fed. The cheapest and fastest way to fatten animals (*and people*) is to serve them corn, corn-fed meat, soy, and sugar. With this combination, we are able to supersize at a faster rate than ever before. And indeed we have!

Summary
Miracle Foods or Poison?

- Is the mass production of inexpensive and imperishable *miracle* foods a blessing or a curse? Many of our miraculous staples are repackaged poisons.

- A huge amount of what we eat comes from corn, corn-fed meat, corn oil, or corn fillers. The corn feeding frenzy is harming our environment and ruining the health of humans and livestock alike.

- Feeding corn to salmon and beef alters their fat composition. Accordingly, corn-fed protein sources do not provide us with the omega-3 fatty acids that we can get from wild-caught or grass-fed sources.

- The development of ammonium nitrates and pesticides has allowed farmers to dramatically increase crop yield. However, these poisons don't just vanish into the soil. They flow into our streams and rivers, polluting everything in their course.

- Like corn, soy is a master of disguise, hidden in countless products.

- Even though soy is heralded as a natural health food, its products are actually some of the most refined and processed foods available.

- Studies have connected soy consumption with goiters, growth problems, amino acid deficiencies, mineral malabsorption, endocrine disruption, and cancer.

- Vegetable oils, such as canola, palm, sunflower, safflower, cottonseed, grapeseed, peanut, soybean, and corn oil are highly processed, unnatural, and unhealthy. The same holds true for the solidified forms as well (i.e., margarine and other fake butter products).

- Unfortunately vegetable oils, like corn and soy, are everywhere, in almost every packaged, manufactured, or fried food out there.

- Canola oil, the star player in this team of oils, is a modified version of rapeseed oil. Rapeseed oil comes from the (inedible) cotton plant. Factories use petroleum solvent under very high temperatures in order to remove the erucic acid (a.k.a. poison) from the soon-to-be canola oil. After more acid, heat, and chemical treatments, the result is finally palatable. Called "low erucic acid rapeseed," or LEAR, this chemical soup was christened canola oil in 1980 as a marketing ploy.

- Although we cannot assume causation, it is interesting to note that the rise of heart disease, diabetes, and obesity over the past century parallels the rise of vegetable oil usage.

- Vegetable oils are high in omega-6's, which are unstable under heat and can cause inflammation, cell mutation, and disease states in the long term.

- Instead of using vegetable oil, cook meals with healthy, stable fats.

- Refined sugar, or sucrose, depletes the body of important vitamins and minerals, including sodium, calcium, magnesium, and potassium.

- Excessive sugar intake eventually affects every organ in the body and causes lethal diseases.

- The best ways to avoid the toxicity of our modern diets is to wash the poisons off your produce, buy organic and local, and avoid imperishable, manufactured products.

~ 9 ~

Superfoods 101

Pollution, toxins, cigarette smoke, radiation, herbicides and pesticides, chemicals in household products and toiletries, psychological stress, lack of sleep, rancid fats—These are just some of the combatants that stealthily attack our health every single day by creating free radicals in our bodies. Remember, free radicals are those unstable molecules that lead to cell damage and cell death and on a bigger scale, speed up the aging process and increase our vulnerability to cancer, heart disease, and other deadly illnesses.

As we've talked about before, free radicals work through oxidation. So the best way to combat their destructive power is by ingesting God's natural antidote: antioxidants.

Exhibit A: The Orange

Besides fiber and calcium, this citrus fruit provides you with a big dose of vitamin C and other antioxidants. When you eat an orange, the antioxidants turn free radicals into unreactive conjugates, which are *not* harmful to us, and thus prevent and even undo damage like cell death, inflammation, and cellular excitation. That's why the orange is a superfood.

Superfoods are foods that are naturally jam-packed with nutrition, relative to their caloric value or size. These high-power foods are not only fully capable of satiating our bodies; they are nature's medicine, packed with vitamins and minerals that heal diseased tissue, build up body structure, decrease inflammation, combat disease, and slow aging.

We can get these necessary vitamins and minerals through one-a-day supplements, right? Surely, we don't have to monitor our superfood intake as long as we have pills. Unfortunately, no. Our colons don't like to accept vitamins and minerals unless they come from a natural source. They insist on the real deal.

The proof is in the statistics. Americans are big fans of taking vitamin supplements. Moreover, processed food products are often enriched with vitamins and minerals. Yet 92 percent of Americans are deficient in one or more vitamins and minerals![1] According to a USDA survey, 75 percent of Americans are not getting enough zinc, 40 percent are not getting enough iron, 70 percent not enough vitamin E, and 37 percent not enough vitamin C.[2]

The scary part is each element does so much for your body that deficiency in even one vitamin or mineral can lead to cellular and molecular dysfunction. For instance, magnesium alone can catalyze over three hundred different biochemical reactions! It shouldn't come as a surprise then that diets deficient in plant foods are connected with many of today's chronic diseases. Strokes, gout, deep vein thrombosis or DVT (blood clots that can travel through the bloodstream and lodge in the lungs, brain, and heart), kidney stones, gallstones, pernicious anemia, hypertension, heart disease, constipation, irritable bowel syndrome, Crohn's disease, tooth decay, autoimmune disorders, and obesity *are all connected to a diet that is low in plant foods.*[3] Eesh!

So let's figure out where and how we can get the necessary vitamins and minerals into our bodies in compact, powerful doses. What should we eat? What are the superfoods in each food group?

Carbohydrate Superfoods

I. Vegetables

- dark, leafy greens: kale, arugula, collard greens, mustard greens, watercress, romaine, red leaf lettuce, spinach, Swiss chard— Usually, it's this category's most pungent and earthy-tasting greens that will carry the most bang for the buck. These dark, leafy greens are valued for their rich content of calcium, B vitamins, vitamin E, vitamin K, potassium, beta-carotene, and chlorophyll. They also contain antioxidants like vitamin C, lutein, and zeaxanthin. The benefits are vast: healthy skin and hair, improved memory, arthritis relief, bone health, improved mood, and improved vascular health.

- cruciferous vegetables: broccoli, cauliflower, brussels sprouts, purple and green cabbage, radishes, bok choy—All are members of the cabbage family. Research is connecting these miraculous antioxidant vegetables with cancer-preventing and even fat-dissolving qualities! In addition, several compounds in these vegetables are linked to the activation of detoxification enzymes. Studies show that, in just three weeks of eating cruciferous vegetables, oxidative stress (which forms free radicals) can be reduced! Interestingly, that same study also showed that supplemental vitamins do not reduce oxidative stress.[4] There's no way around it; you have to eat your veggies.

- roots and tubers: sweet potatoes, turnips, ginger, beets, rutabagas, parsnips, and their relatives carrots, celery, parsley, and fennel—roots contain vitamin A, vitamin C, beta-carotene, minerals, fiber, antioxidants, calcium, and potassium. These vegetables add a healthy, fiber-rich sweetness to our meals. Try substituting your bread, corn, rice, or white potatoes with one of these lower-GI, flavorful, vitamin-rich starches. A sweet potato, for example, takes almost no time to prepare and is rich in vitamins as well as tasty and filling. Ginger is also worthy of special mention. For centuries, Asian cultures have used ginger as a medicinal treatment for arthritis, nausea, and digestive problems. More recently, ginger has been heralded for its metabolism-boosting qualities.[5]

- bulbs: garlic, leeks, onions, shallots—Studies show that diets rich in bulbs may lower one's risk for several types of cancer. Bulbs are also known for their ability to thin mucous and dissolve fats. Additionally, garlic is valued for its antibacterial, antiviral, and anti-inflammatory properties.

- squash: acorn, spaghetti, pumpkin, zucchini, summer, butternut—These brightly colored vegetables impart a naturally sweet taste and are filled with fiber, vitamin A, vitamin C, manganese, magnesium, potassium, selenium, and zinc. They protect against birth defects, promote heart health, and reduce symptoms of asthma and arthritis. Dash some cinnamon or curry on top, and you've got an anti-inflammatory feast.

- fermented vegetables: pickles, sauerkraut, pickled green beans/ onions/beets/cauliflower/asparagus—The process of fermentation requires all the right bacteria, the bacteria that keep our bodies running and are vital to digestive and immune health.

II. Fruits

- blueberries— one of the most powerful antioxidant foods. They contain the substance pterostilbene, which is very efficient at lowering cholesterol. Blueberries are also rich in manganese, anthocyanine, vitamin C, and fiber.

- black currants— full of bioflavonoid antioxidants. These berries contain three times the vitamin C of an orange. Vitamin C keeps your skin looking youthful and baby-soft.

- kiwi— also rich in vitamin C. Moreover, kiwis have six times the potassium of a banana, making them a better choice to prevent muscle cramps or sore muscles after a workout. Kiwi contains lutein as well, which helps prevent macular degeneration (a leading cause of visual problems in the elderly).

- citrus fruits— rich in beta-carotene, folic acid, and vitamin C. Citrus fruits can contain more than 170 different phytochemicals and 60 flavinoids (antioxidant chemicals). Among the benefits are healthy skin, a decrease in free radical formation, and disease-fighting properties. Citrus also provides protection from mouth, throat, and stomach cancer.[6]

- coconut— strengthens the immune system, improves digestion, increases metabolism, helps with weight loss, and improves the function of the nervous system.

- black cherries— great for reducing inflammation, which is important for everyone (inflammation causes disease states) but especially for people with collagen disorders, arthritis, injuries, or cardiovascular disease.

- apples— contain a special pectin fiber that protects the body from pollution and are reported to relieve indigestion, gout, arthritis, and even hangovers. In addition, frequent consumption of apples may lower weight and cholesterol. "An apple a day...," right?

- papaya and guava— high in potassium; vitamins C, A, K, and E; folate; and fiber. Great for digestion, to boot.

- pomegranates (and other intensely colored berries)— extremely high in antioxidants.[7]

Don't hold yourself to this limited list of fruits and vegetables; many of those not listed here have similar health benefits. Eat whatever is fresh and seasonally available. But remember, fruit is nature's dessert. About two servings of fruit gives you all the benefits without a sugar overdose.

III. Herbs and Spices

- Cinnamon, chili peppers, turmeric, garlic, oregano, basil, thyme, ginger, and rosemary are some of the best studied and most valued to date. But the list goes on—tarragon, sage, mint, dill, paprika, parsley, cilantro, curry, cumin ... *All brightly colored, flavor-packed herbs fit our superfood definition to a T.*

- Herbs and spices provide a tremendously sophisticated path toward flavor and satisfaction. As a matter of fact, *they help you reach satiety with far fewer calories than if you were eating bland food.* When you can, use fresh herbs. Otherwise, substitute with dried spices. Once you start cooking, you'll see that it's actually loads of fun to experiment with these different flavors, all the while improving your skin tone and the health of your teeth, nails, and hair.

- Common herbs and spices lower inflammation and thereby benefit all sorts of chronic conditions, such as heart disease, arthritis, diabetes, and cancer. Red pepper, cinnamon, and turmeric are particularly known for their anti-inflammatory properties. Chili peppers—if you can handle them—contain capsaicin, which may lower blood pressure, and dihydrocapsiate, which may boost the frequent consumer's fat-burning capacity. I could write an entire book just about the healing properties of herbs and spices; they are the superfoods of all superfoods.[8, 9]

Fat Superfoods

Think back to "How Our Bodies Use Food" where we learned about essential fatty acids and in particular omega-3's (the kings of nutrition). Here's a summary of what fats do for us:

Fats...

- form the structure of all one hundred trillion cell membranes in our bodies
- affect metabolism and aid in weight maintenance
- control gene function
- reduce inflammation
- help balance blood sugar
- act as our brain's fertilizer, facilitating new cell growth and connections
- play a critical role in brain development, learning, spatial memory, and visual development
- promote joint function and mobility
- improve skin and complexion health
- contribute to positive behavior in children
- boost mood
- are key to hZeart health, mental health, nervous system function, and immune function[10]

The superfats I list below are mostly sources of omega-3's. However, phospholipids and *good* cholesterol are the other fats that boost cell membrane health and brain health. Phospholipids can be obtained from egg yolks, peanuts, lentils, and flaxseeds. And good cholesterol can be obtained from eggs, poultry, and shrimp.[11] Monounsaturated fats are also healthy and are found in nuts, avocados, and flaxseed, as well.

- pecans (the antioxi-*nut*) —Pecans have the highest amount of antioxidants of any nut, over nineteen vitamins and minerals, and beta-sitosterol, which lowers cholesterol.[2, 13]

- brazil nuts—These nuts are high in selenium, a mineral antioxidant that protects the body from the free radicals that can cause heart disease and premature aging.

- walnuts—Walnuts are rich in omega-3 fatty acids and vitamin E. They may help protect against Alzheimer's disease. They also improve cholesterol levels and increase serotonin levels (mood booster). Their plethora of omega-3 fats also contribute to radiant skin and mental acuity.

- olives and olive oil—Olives are another fruit (surprisingly) that are a monounsaturated fat and promote good cholesterol. They contain polyphenols—great antioxidants that help lower blood pressure and prevent cardiovascular disease.

- salmon, especially *wild-caught* salmon—In general, wild-caught fish oils are great sources of omega-3 fats.[14]

- wild game and grass-fed beef—These meats have omega-3's galore.

- seeds, particularly pumpkin and sunflower seeds—Seeds contain protein, fiber, healthy fats, and minerals, such as magnesium, iron, zinc, and manganese. They also contain phytosterols, which are helpful in decreasing cholesterol and boosting the immune system.

- chocolate—Chocolate? A superfood? Well, here's the catch: the cocoa is what makes it super, not all the added sugar. Choose to eat the more flavorful, low-sugar, dark chocolate *in moderation.* Reported benefits include increased blood flow, lowered blood pressure, and decreased risk of stroke. Plus, chocolate releases endorphins that mimic the feeling of falling in love!

- butter, especially from pastured, grass-fed cows—Butter contains fat-soluble vitamins and other nutrients, healthy saturated fat, and a compound called *activator X* that helps prevent disease and improve nutrient absorption.[15]

- avocado—Avocado is primarily a source of monounsaturated fats but an incredibly healthy fat choice. It's also a great source of vitamin E, which prevents the oxidation of LDL (a detrimental triglyceride). Avocados are also high in vitamin B-6, which is crucial for a healthy nervous system. Low levels of vitamin B-6 are associated with depression and chronic fatigue.

Protein Superfoods

Recall that proteins make up enzymes (which initiate every cellular reaction), immune system messengers, hormones, neurotransmitters—in short, proteins make up our bodies. And yet we cannot produce ten of the twenty different amino acids that link together to make proteins. The Biology Project of the University of Arizona explains that "Failure to obtain enough of even 1 of the 10 essential amino acids, those that we cannot make, results in degradation of the body's proteins—muscle and so forth—to obtain the one amino acid that is needed. Unlike fat and starch, the human body does not store excess amino acids for later use—the amino acids must be in the food every day."[16]

Complete protein sources, which provide all the amino acids you need, include the following:

- fish—Seafood contains a great assortment of the essential amino acids, as well as magnesium, selenium, phosphorous, vitamins A and D, and of course, lots of omega-3's. Anchovies are also an excellent source of calcium.[17]

- cottage cheese, preferably whole or 2 percent fat— Besides being an excellent source of protein, *whole-fat* cottage cheese allows our bodies to maximally absorb the calcium it provides.

- Greek yogurt, preferably whole or 2 percent fat—Like cottage cheese, it is low in calories and rich in protein, and it's healthy fat content facilitates calcium absorption.

- eggs—Eggs are an inexpensive, complete protein source and one of the most nutrient-packed foods out there. They are loaded with vitamins and minerals that we often don't get enough of in our daily diets.

- grass-fed, lean/extra-lean meat—Many people think chicken and turkey are the only healthy meat options. On the contrary, we need a variety of lean meats in our diets to achieve optimal health. Red meat provides an array of amino acids that aid in healing small muscular tears—crucial for athletes! It's also an amazing source of iron, which keeps your energy up and helps carry oxygen throughout your body. Since young women are particularly susceptible to iron deficiencies, a regular meal with red meat is a great idea. What's more, lean meats are jam-packed with magnesium (which builds bones), zinc (vital to immune system function), and B vitamins (which boost metabolism, help form red blood cells, aid in converting carbohydrates into fuel, and are crucial to our nervous system).[18]

- legumes—Legumes are not complete protein sources on their own. However, beans of all kinds are rich sources of protein, vitamins, and complex carbohydrates. They supply a huge dose of fiber and contain cancer-fighting antioxidants.

Dairy Superfoods

Dairy products are healthy as long as you stick to low-fat, fat-free, reduced-fat, or skim, right? That's certainly the conventional wisdom. Unfortunately, that is completely misguided thinking.

Skim milk and fat-free yogurt have fewer grams of fat but *more grams of sugar*. Which source of calories is better for you—healthy fat, which keeps you satiated for longer, has enormous health benefits, and doesn't get stored as body fat, or sugar, which is stored as body fat and has no health benefits? This isn't a trick question. It's much better to eat dairy products the way they were intended to be (with fat) than the refined, lower fat but more sugary versions.

This point is underlined by the fact that some of dairy's health perks are lost when the fat is removed. Fat-soluble vitamins, such as vitamins A, K, E, and D, need fat to be absorbed by the body, which is probably why God put the two substances together in the first place.[19, 20]

With our fat-free dairy bias, it makes sense that around 41 percent of Americans are vitamin D deficient.[21] Why does this matter? Because we've learned that vitamin D is *as* important as calcium for maintaining strong, healthy bones. Moreover, it's a natural mood enhancer.

Since we also can get vitamin D from sunlight, scientists went to northern Finland, where the sun barely appears during winter months, to research the importance of vitamin D for our bodies. What they found is this: *vitamin D is vital for every single cell in the body.*

If 41 percent of Americans are deficient, chances are you are too. Talk to your doctor about your vitamin D levels. Since fifteen minutes of sunshine provides us with about 15,000 international units of vitamin D, I'd recommend almost everyone to take 1,000 or 2,000 units per day. If you've had very little exposure to sunshine or you're intolerant to dairy, this is especially important.

Besides vitamin D, dairy provides calcium, vitamin B-2 and B-12, potassium, magnesium, and much more. Again, if you're dairy intolerant, please be conscious of taking in these nutrients from other foods. For example, green, leafy vegetables, seafood, beans, nuts, and seeds can fulfill your body's calcium requirements.

What about dairy superfoods?

- yogurt—As I mentioned in regards to pickled vegetables, fermentation allows for the proliferation of healthy bacteria. Believe it or not, the human body has ten times more bacteria than human cells![22] This symbiotic relationship is actually incredibly important because these microscopic microbes act as our first level of defense against many illnesses. For thousands of years, people took in these friendly bacteria through lots of different sources because they had to pickle anything they wanted to preserve. Today, we have freezers, refrigerators, chemical preservatives, and airtight packages, and as a result, we have almost eliminated fermented foods from our diets. So it's more important than ever to eat yogurt that says on its label "with live active cultures" and "probiotics."

- Frequently eating fermented foods such as yogurt has been shown to improve, or at least relieve, many gastrointestinal disorders (lactose intolerance, candida infections, constipation, diarrhea, colon cancer, inflammatory bowel disease, and *H. pylori* infections to name a few).[23, 24]

- It's a shame, but most people not only take in more sugar by choosing low-fat yogurts; they also shoot themselves in the foot by choosing flavored or sweetened yogurts. *Flavored yogurt is not a health food; it's a dessert.* Don't fall prey to the marketing ploys that make you think yogurt is only edible if it tastes like vanilla pudding. Don't feed into our society's sugar addiction by convincing yourself you can't stomach plain yogurt.

- Addictions never get satisfied. The more sugar you put into your diet, the more you'll want. Instead of giving in to that vicious cycle, why not improve flavor by combining superfoods? Add blueberries or cinnamon to your plain yogurt. Or stir in a drop of honey or a glob of peanut butter. I bet you'll be surprised by how much you like it.

Now you know which foods act as natural antidotes to the external stressors we are plagued with daily. The next step is to stock up your medicine cabinet by going to the grocery store and loading up on avocados, plain yogurt, blueberries, kale, grass-fed meat, and loads of herbs and spices. Maybe your at-home pharmacy will ward off illness so effectively that you'll never have to step foot inside a commercial drugstore again. And at the same time, maybe you'll ward off unhealthy weight gain so effectively you'll never have to go on a diet again.

Summary
Superfoods 101

- Pollution, toxins, cigarette smoke, radiation, herbicides and pesticides, chemicals in household products and toiletries, psychological stress, lack of sleep, and rancid fats all create unstable molecules that lead to cell damage and cell death.

- Antioxidants found in superfoods are the antidotes to this oxidative stress. Whole, natural foods are medicinal and have properties that undo damage from external and internal stressors.

- Supplemental vitamins do not reduce oxidative stress, whether in pills or injected into manufactured foods (as advertisements claim).

- This entire chapter is a concise summary of the nutritional benefits of food. Refer to it as needed, and make sure to consume plenty of foods as they come from the earth in order to improve metabolism and optimize health.

~ 10 ~

Cognitive Therapy

Disordered eating and obesity are not simply behavioral or physiological problems; they are fundamentally psychological as well. For this very reason, any attempt to treat or prevent eating-related illnesses would be incomplete without providing psychological tools for recovery and health. The most important psychological tool is cognitive behavior therapy, or simply cognitive therapy.

Cognitive therapy is a well-accepted form of psychotherapy, essentially a natural but incredibly successful way of transforming your perspective on everything—on yourself, your health, your future, your relationships, your weight... When other forms of treatment fail, or offer only temporary fixes for deep-rooted problems, it can provide long-term success without drugs or invasive medical intervention. In fact, cognitive therapy has been found to be *at least as effective as medication in the long run* for treating people who are prone to worry and depression.[1,] [2] It can be the difference between insecurity and confidence, despair and contentment, even life and death. Most relevant to us, however, is the fact that *cognitive work is a preferred method of treatment for eating problems because of its natural and lifelong curative benefits.*[3]

Here's how it works. The goal is to discover and then eliminate the cognitions that negatively affect mood and behavior. We can then establish a *consistently* positive and healthy psychological state, one that helps us meet the challenges we face, both now and in the future.

In order to start this process, the first step is to identify the negative thoughts that serve as corrosive acid, the so-called "cognitive distortions" that eat away at our happiness and self-esteem. There are three relevant categories of cognitive distortions that people use for their own self-damaging purposes.

1. <u>Automatic negative thoughts:</u> These are the ruinous comments that we repeat in our heads, usually without even realizing it. "I'm so awkward." "I can't do *anything* well." "Could I be any more of an idiot?" These flippant, insulting thoughts chip away at our self-esteem, slowly but surely. In fact, body dissatisfaction is intimately connected to these self-destructive cognitions.

2. <u>Overgeneralizations and distortions:</u> Let's use an example that pertains to food. "Meat contains animal fat. Fat is fattening. I'm never going to eat meat again." That line of thinking is very common, even though it's based on the logical fallacy that eating fats makes you fat. Almost any scenario can be tainted by these kinds of distortions. Consider this statement, for instance: "If I eat anything after 6:00 p.m., it'll go straight to my waist. I won't let myself eat after 6:00 p.m. Ever." That's a distortion. It's not like at 5:50 you're safe, but ten minutes later, you're in danger of spontaneously ballooning out. Finally, here's an overgeneralization that has been the source of a great deal of pain and hurt: "Fat people are lazy and unmotivated. They're fat because they don't take care of themselves." Do you see how traumatizing cognitive distortions can become?

3. <u>Catastrophization:</u> This is where we turn molehills into mountains. Expert catastrophizers have an amazing knack for turning something little, like a four-pound weight fluctuation, into a horrifying calamity.

Different thought patterns have the power to change the course of our lives. With enough self-destructive thinking, we could bring on an anxiety disorder, depression, rage, panic, migraines, insomnia, violence, suicidal thinking, and the list goes on.

But there is a flip side (thank goodness!). We can also use that same tremendous power that we have—the power of sculpting our cognitions—to change our mind-set *for the better.* It's up to each of us. We can choose to let our minds run down that slippery slope of destructive thinking, *or* we can choose to use cognitive therapy to encourage our minds down a different path—the path to health and happiness.

Cognitive Restructuring

Let's break down the steps involved in this therapeutic remodeling tool.

1. Identify destructive thoughts. Is it an automatic negative thought? An overgeneralization or distortion? Or is it catastrophization? Expose these parasitic cognitions for what they are, and then make *them* the objects of contempt instead of yourself.

2. Adopt new thinking patterns. Train your mind just like you would train your body through exercise. Strengthen the neural pathways in your brain that create a positive psyche. Replace degrading self-talk with uplifting self-talk.

3. Force yourself to present the contrasting viewpoint. If you can't see the sunny side to every situation, turn on a lamp. *Find* the bright side. Create it, if you must. Dwell on the positive elements of life, even if they are smaller and more difficult to see, because optimists tend to be happier people, perform better in jobs, and suffer less in the midst of challenges.

Our goal is to harness the incredible power we have at our fingertips—our brainpower—for good rather than self-destruction.

Now, I just said that you need to exercise and train your mind, just like you'd exercise your body at the gym. So let's do an exercise, some mental Tae Bo, if you will.

Think about a horribly embarrassing situation you've experienced or a past mistake that torments you. Conjure up all the shame, humiliation, and self-hate you can muster. Use any or all of the cognitive distortions we've discussed to marinate in your misery.

Not too much fun, right? I'd say it's downright dismal, actually. So then, why do we do it?

The worst kind of tormentor is ourselves. That's why people who are masters at cognitive distortions are some of the most insecure and unhappy people in the world. Facing incessant internal abuse, they become beggars, constantly seeking out external reassurance. Alas, the admiration or validation that they seek will never fully fill the pit created by their own self-destructive thinking.

We never want to put our self-esteem in other people's hands. Think about it. When you encounter competitive or sadistic people, do you think they'll be mindful of the fragility of the human self-esteem? Do you think they'll handle your self-confidence with the utmost care that it deserves? What if they have too many problems of their own to be your constant voice of encouragement? Will they ever be able to fill your neediness, wipe away your insecurity, and heal your wounds?

If only!

No, the only way to protect your self-esteem and your mental health is to take back the power that is undeniably yours: the power to give yourself a sense of self-worth. And then, you must use that power wisely.

Let's go back to that humiliating scenario you just blew out of proportion and do some more mental Tae Bo. This round, I want you to exercise self-construction. Try to undo the shame. Think of as many ways to salvage your wounded spirit as you can. What kinds of cognitions heal your psychological shame and fear?

Careful, though … It's tempting to build yourself up with loads of false truths in an effort to rescue your self-esteem. If you don't know what I mean, just watch an episode of the *Bachelor* or *Bachelorette*; some of the contestants will show you. "I'm so good-looking; these people are just jealous." "They can't handle what a catch I am." "I deserve so much better than everyone around me. I'm too smart to put up with their immaturity." This tactic of self-aggrandizement isn't limited to contestants on the shows though. Anyone can do it, which means some serious self-examination is in order for all of us.

The thing is, putting yourself up on a pedestal is just as dangerous as throwing yourself into the gutter of self-hate. Pedestals are wobbly, and as soon as reality hits, you're going to be knocked right off that lofty perch. And that's a hard fall.

Denial of flaws and narcissistic repairs are not the solution. Acceptance, humor, and love are much safer choices. It's important to be able to laugh at yourself; don't take yourself too seriously. That gives you room for mistakes. Learn to accept imperfections and love the *real* you.

Now I'd like you to answer a few questions in a journal. If you don't consider yourself the journaling type of person, I want to encourage you to give it another shot. Journaling is an incredibly effective way to self-examine, to practice self-love and self-expression in a safe and healthy environment, and to initiate personal growth.

In your journal, please list any cognitive distortions that you have allowed to roam around your brain. Do you distort or exaggerate your problems? If so, how? Describe it in detail. Do you succumb to automatic, negative thoughts? How are these thoughts affecting your sense of self-worth?

Now for the last part of the mental exercise: I want you to tap into the power that you used to resurrect the anxiety from your embarrassing memory and then channel it to work for your advantage. See if you can redirect your brainpower to calm the fear and repair the injured self.

To give you an idea of how this works, let's look at a fictional cognitive distortion and see if we can practice restructuring.

"Leave it to me to find a way to have cellulite on top of cellulite. That's skill, right there. I can't even fit into my clothes anymore. I hate myself."

Now comes the moment of choice. This person could either stop right there and thereby reinforce the insecurities and wounds that lead to destructive behavior, *or* she could say...

"Stop. I'm not going to do this again to myself. With that kind of negative thinking, it's a wonder I can function at all! I know I'm imperfect; I always will be. But the last thing I want to do is abuse myself when I'm already hurting. The person under this exterior of mine is loving and earnest. I want to cherish this person, not destroy her! Honey, you *are* lovable."

Bravo. That's the kind of thought pattern that will pull someone out of an anxiety-provoking, problem-exaggerating, ruminative cycle and reengage the neural pathways that create a calm, content state of mind.

From now on, every time you notice one of those cognitive distortions crawling in through the cracks of your mind, beat it over the head with a figurative baseball bat! You're the exterminator. It's your job to keep your psyche free from those detrimental thoughts.

Self-soothing through cognitive restructuring is a perfect treatment for any type of psychological pain, and in the long run, it sure beats the ice cream sundae cure. But remember that practice makes perfect. Just like with physical training and exercising, you need to build up strength of mind through repetition and perseverance. So keep practicing establishing healthy thought patterns. The reward will be worth it, I promise. Eventually, you will be free to focus on the important issues in life, the things that really matter to you, rather than directing all your energy toward cleaning up emotional toxic spills.

Your Internal Parent Voice

All of us naturally internalize the voices of our past caregivers, either copying or rebelling against them, depending on how they affected us. If we were neglected as children, for instance, we might either continue the pattern through self-neglect or overcompensate through self-indulgence. If we were verbally abused as children, we might engage in self-abuse or conversely, in egotistical self-praise.

The good news is you aren't necessarily doomed to imitating or rebelling against the kind of parenting you received as a child. No matter what your upbringing was like, you can ask yourself, "What type of internal parent voice do I want going forward?" Through cognitive restructuring, you can establish a healthy internal parent voice that encourages personal growth.

What would the ideal parent look like?

Well, he or she wouldn't succumb to the temptation of overindulgence, because real love provides discipline, not just pampering. Excessive gifts of decadent food, undeserved praise, intense experiences, material possessions, and behavioral leniency perpetuate immaturity and bad habits.

Sadly, too many people in our society are accustomed to this type of parenting. Why? Well, studies show that overindulgence is connected with prior abuse and neglect.[4] Parents who are stretched too thin, trying to balance responsibilities at work and home, feel guilty that they cannot give their children the attention and time they deserve. So they make up for it by spoiling them. The result is a demographic of people who have grown to expect immediate gratification and as a consequence, lack the ability to discipline themselves.

This attitude of entitlement can influence every sphere of life, from the political to the personal. *When it comes to eating habits in particular, our impulsive, self-spoiling tendencies mean that we cater to our taste buds' never-ending demands.* It's as if we're suddenly rendered powerless when our sweet tooth calls or when we have a craving for something. But we're *not* powerless. We can use discipline to act as a respectable, reasonable, responsible human being. Plus on an intellectual level, we know better than to give in to our destructive impulses. All we have to do is give wisdom the reins instead of our pleasure-seeking urges.

Knowledge + Discipline = Success

It's a two-part formula. Having one without the other doesn't cut it. This is blatantly obvious when we consider the amount of nutritional information that is accessible to our society. Health books, blogs, magazines, apps—you name it! But even if these information sources get it right (since so many of them are contradictory), knowledge isn't enough. No amount of nutritional education can save our society from its obesity and eating disorders crises unless we recognize and address the fact that a lack of discipline is as much to blame as a lack of knowledge.

Consider the following thought pattern:

"I'm hungry, or maybe I'm just bored or tired. Either way, I want something and I want it now. Hmmm … that chocolate cake looks amazing. And I deserve it! Yup, I'm gonna have it. I mean, YOLO! No regrets."

For those of you who aren't familiar with the meaning of YOLO (my daughter only recently enlightened me), it's the "You only live once" motto that describes our modern society perfectly. It's a terribly dangerous idea, actually; it gives us license to do anything we want, no matter how detrimental. "No regrets" is a similarly common mantra, with similarly hedonistic effects.

You only live once, so you might as well enjoy every minute. Who gives a—about long-term effects? Live in the moment. Carpe diem. Seize the day. Live like there's no tomorrow. The clichés go on and on.

Yes, we want to enjoy every moment of today but not in ways that sabotage our ability to enjoy tomorrow. How will you carpe diem when you're diabetic or suffering from metabolic syndrome? Do you think your elderly self will be mad at her former self for disregarding *her* wishes to enjoy the moment too?

Why not look at it this way: YOLO. You only live once, so treat that life as the sacred gift it is, in its *entirety*, not just for the time being. Seize the day by making smart choices. Then when you're lying on your deathbed and you've enjoyed a very long, good-quality life, you will really be able to look back and say, "No regrets."

Let's reconsider the thought pattern from earlier:

"I'm hungry, or maybe I'm just bored or tired. Either way, I want something and I want it now. Hmmm ... that chocolate cake looks amazing. And I deserve it! Yup, I'm gonna have it."

How is this different from what a two-year-old would do? Like parenting a toddler, it will require constant attention to bring the immature, overindulged part of you to maturity with a loving internal parent voice. Thankfully as children mature, they take less and less constant attention. You just have to walk the walk until it becomes your gait, your lifestyle.

"Yes, I am tired. I had a really hard day, and I need to vent." *(I go stage right and vent, vent, vent to myself.)* "Okay ... What else do I need?"

"Well, I'm still hungry!" *(Sob, sob ...)*

"Hey, sweetie, I have something fabulous for you: a gorgeous, towering, juicy, crunchy, vibrant-green magic wand, also known as celery. We can decorate it with a spoonful of peanut butter or garlic hummus, or we can get creative and wrap it in a slice of smoked turkey and Swiss cheese. Notice the fabulous colors and cherish the crunch. It is medicine for your body. Enjoy it slowly and savor the flavors of gourmet living."

Laugh all you want at my celery imagery; I won't be offended! But don't discard the main point of the example. A truly loving parent needs to take over. A brilliant caregiver can use the power of cognitive restructuring to bring about medicinal treatment for a beleaguered body and brain and can even create motivation and excitement over disciplined living.

I must point out, however, that there is a difference between a good parent and a slave-driver. If you impose rules on yourself through punishment, shaming, or self-abuse, you are simply resorting to cognitive distortions again. Worse, you're giving your inner child reason for retaliation, revenge, and passive-aggressive behavior, all of which hamper progress.

The quality of your internal parent voice will determine how successful you can be with any endeavor, whether it is your education, your job, or your weight management. It is easy to submit to the wise, caring parent who guides you daily through a process of high yet realistic expectations, disciplined structure, and loving correction.

While I'd love to claim these ideas as my own, they are far from novel. In fact, two and a half millennia ago, Plato and Aristotle told us two very relevant things:

1. There are three parts of the human soul.[5, 6] The first responds to basic desires and survival needs. The second uses reason to discern right from wrong. And the third? The third part acts. To Plato and Aristotle, the human soul is only properly functioning when the reasoning part is in charge of the other two. An excellent human, then, is one whose reason and wisdom rule over his or her basic desires. Now that you know their conception of human excellence, I have a riddle for you: *A slice of cheesecake and a slice of cheese are placed in front of Aristotle and Plato. Which do they choose?* (This is true ancient philosophy, obviously.)

2. According to Aristotle, humans have the ability not to only become better at making wise choices (through education) but also to train our emotions and impulses![7] "How?" you ask. Through practice. We become brave by acting bravely and kind by acting kindly. Thus, we can be "made perfect by habit."[8] Now, habit-forming takes—you guessed it—discipline. But Aristotle's view that we can train our impulses and desires gives us wonderful hope. Through practice, we can retrain our tendency to succumb to our taste buds' demands, and eventually, it will become natural for us to follow wisdom rather than momentary pleasures.

As for me, I trust the ancients. And you? Will you sacrifice hedonistic pleasures for greater rewards? Will you set up expectations for achievement? Will you adhere to a disciplined, structured life? Will you admire and respect yourself for your selfless sacrifices more than you do for your selfish endeavors? If we truly desire character strength, health, and wisdom, we must become disciples of discipline. Excellence will follow.

Summary
Cognitive Therapy

- Cognitive therapy is one of the most effective forms of treatment for eating disorders, depression, and anxiety.

- The first step in doing cognitive therapy is to identify automatic negative thoughts, overgeneralizations/distortions, or tendencies toward catastrophization. With this insight, you can correctively steer yourself into positive thinking patterns.

- Narcissistic praise is a type of positive thinking based on lies. Rather than leading to recovery, it only delays character development and progress. Dare to be truthful in your self-reflection.

- One of the best ways we can love ourselves is through discipline. Knowledge + discipline = success.

- It is crucial to learn what it means to have a healthy internal parent voice. Practice listening to yourself. Learn how to vent in safe ways, to comfort yourself when suffering, and to pamper yourself in productive ways that lead to health.

~ 11 ~

Practice Makes Perfect— Meal Diary and Journaling

Journaling is a tool widely used in eating disorders programs. However, journaling is a great activity for pretty much anyone, so don't let an apparent lack of eating problems keep you from journaling. We could all benefit from an opportunity to practice self-examination, self-expression, and self-love.

So let's get started! The structure of the type of journaling I outline here forces you to rethink and reform behavioral issues while confronting deeper psychological patterns. Furthermore, it helps you set your intentions and keeps you focused.

In a spare spiral notebook, make three columns on the left page. Label the headers "Meal Plan," "Meal Journal," and "Meal Diary."

- The meal plan column should be a blueprint for your ideal food intake for the day. Write this each morning or at the start of the week. Your meal plan should represent a variety of foods that appeal to your taste buds; it should provide your body with what it physically needs for optimal function; it must include the foods that are reasonably available to you; and it should contain food that you can make yourself, so that you don't necessarily need to rely on someone else for success. If you don't do the cooking at home and have no freedom to determine what's on the menu, you might want to write down food groups rather than specific dishes.

- The meal journal column is for you to document what you actually ended up eating. This end-of-the-day record will be used to identify your weaknesses and strengths in addressing your physiological needs. Highlight any starvation/restriction periods that may have set you up for a binge or, conversely, any bingeing episodes that set you up for a desire to restrict calories later.

- Use the third column, the meal diary, to briefly describe the situations and emotions that surrounded the eating experience. This is your opportunity to learn about your psychological issues. Be bold and insightful as you journal.

Since we need to have plenty of space for the evaluation of thoughts, moods, and other issues, the opposite page will be reserved for elaboration. Label this section simply "Journal." This is where you get to pour out all the emotional issues that you're facing. Use this page as your go-to place for putting words to whatever you may have, in the past, acted out through destructive eating patterns.

No one needs to see this journal, so be honest. Here, you are safe to get rid of anger, rebellion, and pain. Take the opportunity in this section to be authentic, to vent, to repent, and to practice grace and unconditional love with yourself.

Nevertheless, this section is also your opportunity to see where you may be playing the victim role and failing to take responsibility for your shortcomings. The purpose of journaling is full disclosure, which allows us to see our own failings so that we can push on toward success. Dare to be transparent with yourself.

Eve's Meal Diary and Journal

To give us an idea of how to use a meal diary and journal, we're going to have Eve, a fictional friend, show us how it's done. Take it away, Eve!

Time	Meal Plan	Meal Journal	Meal Diary
7:00 a.m.	1 cup steel-cut oats with blueberries, 2 hard-boiled eggs, a cup of coffee with some half-and-half	1 cup steel-cut oats with blueberries, 2 hard-boiled eggs, a cup of coffee with some half-and-half	Proud that I followed my meal plan to the T, but hating how full I feel. Not used to eating breakfast.
12:00 p.m.	Open-faced tuna-and-cheese sandwich (on 1 slice of whole wheat toast), Greek salad with romaine lettuce, feta cheese, kalamata olives, tomatoes, onions, sunflower seeds, and lightly sprinkled olive oil + balsamic vinegar for dressing	Greek salad with iceberg lettuce, feta cheese, olives, tomatoes, and olive oil + balsamic vinegar for dressing	Cut down on lunch since I felt grossly full in the morning. Didn't have all the ingredients for the salad in the house, but I did the best I could.
3:30 p.m.	bowl of berries and 2 percent cottage cheese		Trying not to think about food, but getting so hungry and tired from long shift.
4:00 p.m.		2 double-fudge chocolate-chip cookies	I caved. Don't even wanna talk about it.
6:30 p.m.	Baked salmon with dill, lemon, and olive oil, ½ cup quinoa with chopped onions and peppers, asparagus cooked in coconut oil with salt and pepper	half of a piece of salmon, some asparagus, and a glass of wine	Tried to get back on track with small, healthy dinner. And boy, did I need that glass of wine.
8:30– 9:00 p.m.		caramel kettle corn and peanut M&Ms	Wayyyyyy too much of this junk while watching TV. I did not mean for that to happen. Feeling like a failure.

Journal

Whew, I'm thankful this day is over. I blew it. What on earth happened to me?

The whole day began with me feeling too full (and fat) since I forced myself to eat breakfast for once. It's gonna take me a while to accept the idea that fiber and bulk eaten earlier in the day will stave off my appetite later and crank up my metabolism. I know it's supposed to help me maintain a healthy weight in the long run, but it's just completely counterintuitive when I feel like I've got a food-baby for the first half of the day.

Logically, I decided to hold back on what I ate for lunch then. I told myself I'd get back on track for a nice dinner with the fam. At first, I felt totally fine. But by the time it hit 4:00 p.m., I was absolutely <u>starving</u>. And of course there were these gooey, chocolatey cookies in the nurses' lounge—right at my fingertips. Staring me in the face. I couldn't stop myself! I gobbled down two before I knew it. For a brief, fleeting moment, I felt relief, happiness, comfort, and a rush of energy. But already by the time I walked out of the nurses' lounge, all of that was replaced with shame and disgust with myself.

I immediately vowed to go for a run after work … but then I remembered the chapter I read on using exercise as a way of "undoing" calories or punishing your-self … and I decided I didn't want to feed into a bulimic pathology. I'm not saying that I'm bulimic. No way. But I can't deny that exercise is my "go-to" way to purge, to get rid of the calories I eat.

I tried to get back on track at dinner; I really did. I cooked my husband and two kids a very healthy salmon, quinoa, and asparagus dinner, and I ate a smaller portion than everyone else. But, of course, they weren't used to such a healthy dinner, so when we were watching TV later, they pulled out the popcorn and peanut M&Ms. I guess I hadn't felt all that satisfied with my tiny dinner either, so while I was distracted by Netflix, I just kept reaching for what was in front of me. Who knows how much of that junk I ended up eating? All I know is that the bowls were totally empty by the end of the episode. And my guilt and frustration were higher than ever.

Ughhhhhh. I don't want to force myself to follow these stupid rules for healthy eating when all I do is buck them and then feel guilty afterward. More than any-thing, I don't want to do this useless meal plan anymore! It almost seems like it brings out the worst in me—my rebellion and my anger and self-loathing.

So yes, I ate two cookies and a bunch more junk food at night. But can you blame me? I'm an overworked nurse and mom. Eighty percent of my day is already devoted to doing things for other people. Giving and giving and giving myself. I have so little in life that is ... just for me.

Huh. It's interesting reading this and hearing myself trying to justify and explain away my behavior. Who am I trying to fool? Myself?

I really did want to give this meal plan a shot, and now I just hate myself for not having any willpower. But I don't want to keep doing this. I'm so sick of the endless cycle—eating sugary junk and then having this obligation to starve myself or to exercise hanging over my head. And it doesn't even work in the end! I don't have energy or feel good about myself with these patterns. I definitely don't gain better self-esteem or a more positive body image. I don't really achieve anything.

If I'm perfectly honest though, I don't know if I can break the pattern. I'm too afraid. What's wrong with me? I'm afraid to trust the advice of these so-called "experts" on nutritional science. I know what I'm supposed to do. But I don't want to put my weight in their hands. I want to stay within my comfort zone, with what I already know—exercising and restricting calories. I'm afraid to give up my control.

Hmmmm ... so I guess that's my real reason for restricting and exercising. It's a way for me to feel in control.

So the next question is why do I rebel in the first place?

I think I've got a lot of deep resentment—resentment over the fact that I've always had to please everyone but myself. Maybe the pleasing, submissive smile I put on for the world is just a facade; it's not the real me. I don't really want to be so passive and pleasing and sacrificial, especially since I don't feel that way inside.

Wait ... I think I get it.

The two cookies don't just represent my sweet tooth. They represent one single, precious moment of not having to be perfect and pleasing and sacrificial. They are my way of giving in to myself.

What if I wasn't so pleasing all the time?

Well, I don't think people would like me then. I'm not gorgeous or funny; I was never popular growing up. Underneath my need to control and be perfect for everyone is really my fear that others will see my vulnerability and inadequacy and ... hate it as much as I do.

Wow. This is really, really hard to admit to myself.

I feel so depressed and exposed. Raw. What's left under this mask of perfection is just little old me. I have to try so hard to be worthy of love. Shouldn't I be able to receive love for just being _me_?

Does anyone love me like that? Do I let anyone love me like that?

I don't like to think about how many ways I chain myself to maintaining this perfect, in-control persona. In order for me to create some authentic self-esteem,

I'm going to have to risk losing my image. Be vulnerable. Show the world the real me—and learn to love the real me.

Huh ... If I hadn't written down the fears that are behind giving in to the two cookies, I bet I'd never have had the chance to realize how much I fear failure and my own inadequacies.

Okay, so instead of those stupid cookies, what did I really need in that moment? Ummmm ... I needed a nap, a massage, a talk with my best friend, a moment alone in my room with my music ... I guess there are a lot of things that could have filled the same role that the cookies did.

I know that periodic indulgence is part of the health that I am striving to achieve. But indulgence shouldn't be a momentary lapse of judgment, a rebellious expression of my autonomy, or a pathetic form of self-care. There are better ways to indulge and better ways to show myself love.

So what am I going to do differently tomorrow? Well, first ... I won't let myself freak out by feeling full after breakfast. I'll have healthy snacks throughout the day so I never become starving and overly tired and vulnerable to giving in to my sweet tooth. (I wonder how long it's going to take for me to lose my sweet tooth? If I cut it out completely to break my sugar addiction, it better not take too long ... I'm sick of craving sweets this much. It makes everything so much harder!)

After work, I'll treat myself to a half hour of me time. I'll do something because I want to, not because I feel I need to. Maybe I'll take a nap or take a bath. Those are safe ways for me to listen to my body and remove myself from that insatiable need to please everyone else. If I set this up as my reward, maybe I won't feel deprived, and I won't be indulging in ways that pack on the pounds. You know what? I'm even gonna try doing yoga tomorrow morning instead of my usual hour-long run. I could use that therapeutic relaxation. Plus, the gentle exercise will get me moving without setting my body up with a huge calorie deficit for the rest of the day.

Huh. I'm actually excited about this! Haha. That is <u>not</u> what I expected coming into this journaling thing.

This is going to be good. I'm ready for this kind of change. Let's do this!

****

What will you discover through the journaling process? Your thoughts might look very different than Eve's on paper. Perhaps you don't struggle with immense guilt over your eating patterns. In fact, you might even delight in giving yourself exactly what you want, when you want it. You might be more like Hillary …

Hillary's Journal

I could never give up sweets. Seriously I don't even know how people manage to resist temptations. I simply can't.

Frankly, I wouldn't even want to be a health nut. I see too many people out there living lives of obsessive, controlled frustration ... What is life about if not a little wine, a bubble bath, a day at the beach, a dangerously naughty dessert? It's those wicked indulgences that make life worthwhile.

How sad and pathetic life would be if I became one of those busybody, anal Goody Two-shoes! Especially when it comes to eating. Celery is nasty green hay. Sugar-free, natural yogurt tastes like vomit. Vegetables are disgusting unless it's, like, green beans in one of those yummy baked casseroles with cream of mushroom soup and the fried onions on top ...

I could read endlessly about "nutritional science," and it would all sound fine and dandy for some people. Just not me. I'll leave it to the knitted-clothes-wearing, unshaved-armpit, vegan, hippie weirdos. I'll applaud them from the sidelines as I savor a piece of exquisitely sumptuous gluten-filled, sugar-laden apple pie. Mmmmmmm.

****

In case you haven't already guessed this yourself, Hillary's chances of progress are low. She doesn't *want* to change. No amount of nutritional education is going to help her. She's on the fast track to diabetes, heart disease, and obesity.

Notice how her journaling never got to the point where she was calling herself out on her pathological thinking patterns. Like a child who won't mature into adulthood, Hillary takes pleasure in self-indulgence and doing exactly what she wants. If I could give Hillary some advice, it would go something like this:

"Hillary, your only hope is to work on this cognitively. In other words, you have to change your *thought patterns* in order to change your *emotions* in order to change your *behavior*. How? Like this: Train yourself to think of those 'disgusting' vegetables as life-giving, healing, medicinal, vibrant, and flavorful treats. Practice considering that bowl of sugar-free, natural yogurt as creamy, silky, indulgent, complex, and wickedly smooth ambrosia.

"Use the power of your mind. It's the greatest tool we are given. The power *is* in your hands. Don't let yourself get away with lies like

'I *can't* give up sweets.' Be real with yourself—of course you can. You just don't *want* to give up sweets. But you *would* want to reject them point-blank if you trained yourself to think of them as the addictive, disease-creating, artificial, chemical-ridden poison that they are.

"Change the associations with food that you've fabricated in your mind. Desserts will no longer signify comfort or celebration; they'll represent a lack of self-care, a loss of self-respect, a disregard for the one beautiful body you were given on this earth. Health foods, in contrast, will signify true self-love and the gift of a long life of vitality."

It could be that you are nothing like Eve or Hillary. In fact, you could be closer to the other end of the spectrum. Perhaps, through your meal diary and journal, you will discover that you get your sense of self-worth by staying skinnier than everyone else. Perhaps your journaling will reveal that you take pride in being able to do something most people struggle tremendously with—keeping your weight very low. Perhaps your journaling will look more like Matt's. Matt is a young college student and star cross-country runner who thrives off of people's comments on his physical appearance and holds himself to impossibly high standards in all that he does, including the way he eats.

Matt's Meal Diary and Journal

Time	Meal Plan	Meal Diary	Meal Journal
7:30 a.m.	Steel-cut oats with cheese and 3 scrambled eggs, coffee with whole milk	Steel-cut oats mixed with eggs and cheese and a cafe au lait. 8 oz. water	Easy. I eat this breakfast every day. Perfect kick-starter
10:30 a.m.	Apple with peanut butter	Apple with peanut butter, another glass of water	Feeling good as usual. Already excited for lunch, though.
12:30 p.m.	Loaded turkey sandwich, salad, and milk	Same	Do people really have a hard time following through with this Meal Plan stuff?
3:30 p.m.	Plain yogurt with pineapple, flax seed, and walnuts	Protein bar	Had to grab this on the fly before track practice
7:00 p.m.	Chicken, asparagus, salad, and sweet potato	Chicken, asparagus, salad, and sweet potato with a little bit of butter and cinnamon. Lots of water.	It makes me happy knowing that I'm improving my athletic performance by fueling my body optimally. Colorful, nutritious... great meal.
9:00 p.m.		Seltzer water.	I'm hungry again but I know I shouldn't eat at night. Seltzer water will help me feel full. Obviously, self-control is not a problem for me.
11:00 p.m.			I can't wait for breakfast...

Following my meal plan was easy. I mean, self-control has never been an issue for me. It's what makes me excel and stand out. The only thing I'm wondering is if I should tweak my plan at all... If guys can have as low as 5% body fat, there has to be a way I can get there. I'll make it happen.

I know I'm not supposed to, but I secretly love watching the numbers on the scale go down. I get a thrill out of sculpting my body and seeing its muscle definition. Even the sweat and soreness after a workout give me a sense of accomplishment. It's like a delicious, addictive high that I crave.

But I can't tell anyone this. People would think I'm crazy; they wouldn't understand. We live in this messed-up society where normal = overweight. So of course they don't want me to be thin. But I don't want to be normal, either. I do not want to be like them.

Eesh, that sounded way more judgmental than I intended. Do I really think I'm better than everyone else because of my body? Is this really the way I make myself feel important, attractive, special? Isn't there more to me than my ability to not eat or to work out? That seems a pretty flimsy and sad source of self-worth. I <u>hope</u> I'm worth more than that ...

Take away all my perfectionistic organizing and planning, and who am I? Maybe I'm no different than anyone else, after all. Maybe I'm average, insignificant, or even... not as good. Ouch. That's my greatest fear.

The perfect standard that I hold myself to — somehow it makes me who I am. It defines me; it shapes me, leads me to be better, and ultimately, controls me. I mean, no. I control it. Wait... What do I mean? Was that some kind of Freudian slip? Does it control me???

Agh — that's scary. In a way, yes, it does have control over me. My quest for perfection is never satisfied.

Where did I get this need to be the best, the most stellar student and athlete, the person who never slips up? I have to admit, it's exhausting. And it reflects itself in my overly strict and ritualistic eating habits.

If I'm honest with myself, I can tell the way I think about food, my weight and my self-esteem aren't normal, or healthy for that matter. That's the last thing I want to confess, but it's the truth. I'm enslaved by the rules around eating that I impose upon myself. How can I be rid of these shackles? What would it look like to give myself some grace with my eating habits, and in life in general?

Like freedom, I guess. Do I have the courage to embrace that freedom, though?

****

We all have our own monsters to confront, our own stories to tell. What's your story? Where will your journaling take you? Will you commit to unearthing your truths and correcting your cognitive distortions, whatever they may be?

As you engage in this journaling practice, I hope that you can love yourself enough to mirror back interest, delight, love, and kind words. I hope that you can love yourself enough to be honest and insightful, to find out who you truly are. I hope that you can love yourself enough to strive for more, to take the harder road of a disciplined, purposeful life—one that is full of challenges and full of progress.

~ 12 ~

Final Tips for Success

The goal of this book is to equip you with all the knowledge you need to make healthy choices for the rest of your life. The key word is *choices*. I don't want you to have to live according to somebody else's rules—whether they come from a diet book, the FDA, or a weight-loss program. You deserve to fashion your diet based on a combination of your own preferences and what you know to be healthy. That's what I wish for you. So rather than giving you rules to live by, calories to count, or a list of dos and don'ts, I am going to wrap up this book by providing you with some final tips for healthy living. You don't have to listen to me. Decide for yourself! I promise to always provide *the why* behind my advice so you can fully realize your potential as an individual and an educated consumer.

- Eat three complete meals per day (and one or two snacks, depending on activity level).

    The Why: People lose more body fat when they divide their calories up throughout the day. One study involving two groups of male, Japanese, professional boxers exemplified this fact.[1] The first group ate 2,500 calories per day in only two large meals. The other group also ate 2,500 calories per day, but they split them up over six meals. Which group do you think lost more body fat? Answer: The second group did! Eating the *same amount of calories per day*, they lost significantly more weight, simply because their intermittent, small meals kept their metabolism running all day long.

Warning: The danger with this strategy is that the more times you eat every day, the more opportunities there are to overeat. Self-control is key in order to make sure the total amount of calories per day remains the same.

- Carry healthy snacks with you wherever you go.

    The Why: Snacks keep the hunger monster at bay. Low-sugar/high-protein bars, whole fruits, cut veggies, nuts, natural meat jerky, cheese sticks, yogurt pots—having the right food available prevents emergency mouthfuls of whatever junk food you can lay your hands on. Sadly, it's easier to find bakery items, bags of chips, and candy on the street than healthy snacks, so if you know you're going to be out and about all day, make sure you're prepared ahead of time.

- When eating, sit down at a table with a plate and silverware.

    The Why: Though this sounds like a frivolous thing to include, it helps people monitor what they're eating. Eating out of a bag of popcorn or a jar of peanuts makes it all too easy to mindlessly grab handful after handful of food. Plus, it's important to make meals full, satisfying experiences, and this is achieved more easily when people are intentional and mindful about how they are eating.

- Eat meals with people whenever possible, for similar reasons as above.

    The Why: Meals should be associated with rest, relaxation, social connectedness, enjoyment, and nourishment.

- Eat slowly over a twenty- to thirty-minute period.

   The Why: It takes twenty minutes for the body's sensors to register food quantity and quality. Your brain can tell you how much food your body needs, but you have to give it the chance to do its accounting job accurately. Besides, the slower you eat, the more you get to savor flavors and enjoy table conversation.[2, 3]

- Eat the majority of your calories in the first half of the day.

   The Why: A study looking at the thermic effect of food found that we burn more calories in the morning than in the evening.[4] It makes sense—our bodies have all day to burn off the food that we eat in the morning, whereas after dinner, people usually cease their activity. One of the very best ways to lose weight is to make sure you eat lightly at night and wake up hungry for a good breakfast the next day.

- Eat the majority of your carbohydrate calories (calories from whole grains, fruit, etc.) early in the day.

   The Why: For similar reasons as above. Remember, the body stores any carbs that it doesn't immediately use as fat. Don't give it the chance to do that to you. Since you are unlikely to burn many calories after dinner, this final meal of the day should primarily consist of lots and lots of vegetables, a good protein source, and some healthy fats.

- Include a fasting period in your twenty-four-hour day. Best strategy: Eat your dinner in the early evening, and don't eat again until the next morning.

   The Why: Here's a study involving three groups of mice on three different diets. The first group of mice ate normal chow. The second group ate rich, high-fat food whenever they wanted it throughout the day. The last group of mice ate the *same amount* of high-fat food with the *same amount* of calories, but here's the key: they only ate it during the eight hours of the day during which they were active. For eight hours, these mice probably ate a bit, went on their little treadmill wheels, sewed some clothes for Cinderella, and then ate a bit more. Then, for the next sixteen hours, they fasted. The result? These mice stayed leaner than those who had the *exact same diet* but ate throughout the entire day. In fact, they were just about as healthy as the group 1 mice, who weren't eating high-fat foods. But those unfortunate mice who ate their high-fat diet over the course of a 24-hour cycle (without a fasting period) became obese and developed high cholesterol, high blood sugar, metabolic problems, and fatty livers.[5]

• When food shopping, examine nutrition labels for protein, fat, sugar, and fiber content.

The Why: You want to learn the truth about the food you're consuming and cut through the marketing ploys that make unhealthy foods sound healthy. 100-calorie packs, SkinnyCow ice cream, diet sodas, Odwalla and Naked juice/smoothies, coconut water, vitaminwater®, cereal bars, meal bars, multigrain/whole wheat/heart healthy carbohydrates, non-fat/low-fat/sugar-free desserts, sweetened coffee drinks... when you spot these products, you should see a big red *WARNING, WARNING* flash before your eyes. They are examples of some of the most prominent outrageous seductions in the food industry. Advertising tactics might fool your brain, but they won't fool your body; regardless of what the label says, 36 grams of sugar in a so-called *healthy* beverage will still pack on the pounds.

• Aim to find carbohydrates with at least as many grams of fiber as sugar.

The Why: This will help you stay on the lower end of the glycemic index spectrum. For instance, in General Mills'

Cinnamon Toast Crunch cereal, there are ten grams of sugar and only one gram of fiber. Not the right ratio at all. But in Kashi's GoLean Original cereal, there are six grams of sugar and ten grams of fiber! Jackpot!

- If you can't recognize or pronounce many of the ingredients on the nutrition label, put that puppy back on the shelf.

   The Why: The grocery store is meant to supply you with food, not a chemical soup. So only buy *food*. Skip the chemicals!

- Make naturally colorful meals.

   The Why: A meal that contains an array of colors (from nature, not food dye!) reflects the vast array of nutrients it provides. For instance, a meal of chicken, mashed potatoes, and iceberg lettuce looks bland. Use this as a sign that you need to up the nutritional quality of what you're eating. In contrast, a meal of chicken with sage, sweet potato with butter and salt, and a spinach salad with tomatoes, chopped onions, and sliced avocado is as wonderful for your eyes as it is for your health.

Lastly, I want to address an obstacle that prevents many people from adopting a healthy diet: cost.

It's true that eating organic, local, and fair-trade health foods can be expensive, and shopping at stores like Whole Foods can cost a pretty penny. But choosing a healthy lifestyle doesn't have to break the bank.

How to Eat Healthily on a Tight Budget

- Choose superfoods that are in season.

   Keep an eye out for reasonably priced fresh produce as it goes in and out of season. If you wanna be a true hipster, you could always grow your own herbs in a windowsill or vegetables in a backyard garden.

- Shop at local farmers markets whenever possible.

   Not only will you save yourself money, but you'll also be using your buying power to support local/fair-trade producers instead of big ag companies that monopolize the food industry and may or may not have ethical production practices.

- Buy staple foods and foods with a long shelf life in bulk.

   Places like Costco and Sam's Club help you save money on large quantities. Even if you're not cooking for a huge party or multiple kids, you can buy foods that don't go bad quickly (coconut flour/oil, olive oil, onions, eggs, oranges, cheese, nuts, etc.) and save the excess for later.

- Some healthy foods are consistently cheap and can form a large part of your grocery list if need be.

   Cabbage, peanuts, chicken, legumes, eggs, cucumbers, carrots, apples, oranges, cheese, cottage cheese, and natural peanut butter are all nutritious and typically inexpensive.

- Cook big pots of chili, soups, and stews.

   This is an incredibly helpful way to cut down on costs. Plus, there will be plenty of leftovers to enjoy—no extra money or work required. Moreover, soups and stews can be especially nutritious because all the nutrients are retained in the liquid. This is not true for other methods of cooking vegetables, which cause some of the nutrients to break down or leak out. (This is also a reason not to overcook your veggies!)

- Use a Crock-Pot to make a tough, less expensive cut of meat taste delicious.

   Cut off the major fat, and let it simmer all day in a Crock-Pot with a fourth of a cup of water and seasonings. Try shredding the meat with a fork; it ends up like pulled pork.

So there are, in fact, great ways to eat right without breaking the bank. Like anything else, it just takes learning!

Take the Wheel in Your Life

Congratulations! You did it! You now have all the tools you need for living a healthy and rich life.

Just think how far you've come … First, you learned how pervasive our society's eating problems are; we truly do live in a disordered eating society. Then, you became an expert on why diets don't work, and you can now attest to the fact that diets are the gateway drug for dangerous and lifelong eating problems, even life-threatening eating disorders. In fact, you learned enough about eating disorders to be able to identify the signs and symptoms in yourself and in the people you care about. You have joined the ranks of those who can champion this immeasurably important battle against disordered eating and full-fledged eating disorders.

And that's not all. You understand the vital science of how our bodies use food. You know how protein, carbohydrates, and fats break down in the body. This understanding is the framework with which you are empowered to make wise decisions about what to eat.

What's more, you can even discern between low- and high-quality carbohydrates, using the glycemic index. Like knowing the difference between low- and high-quality fuel at the gas station, this gives you the ability to choose the best types of fuel to fill your body with.

As for exercise, you've got that covered too. Freed from the shackles of obsessive and torturous workout regimens, you get to exercise in ways that are enjoyable and rejuvenating. After all, you know that excessive exercise can actually backfire on the best of intentions when it comes to weight loss.

After reading "The Skinny on How to Stay Lean," you know better than to be fooled by the overly simplified meal plans that have morphed into various geometric shapes over the past century—from "The Basic Seven" to the old food pyramid, the new food pyramid, and now the MyPlate diet. Remember that there's no perfect formula, but it's good to stay within these ballpark ranges: 35 to 45 percent low-GI carbs + 25 to 35 percent protein + 30 to 40 percent healthy fats = 100 percent satisfaction.

By now, you also know the scary truth about soy, corn, vegetable oils, and sugar. These foods are everywhere in the American diet, and their damage to our bodies and to the agriculture industry cannot be overstated.

On the opposite end of the spectrum, superfoods emerge as our natural antidotes and life-giving sources of energy. But I'm just preachin' to the choir. You know all about the benefits of yogurt, blackberries, arugula, herbs and spices, grass-fed meat, and nuts.

Perhaps most important of all, you're now aware that disordered eating is every bit as much of a psychological issue as it is a physiological issue. Our society cannot hope to recover from its eating disorders and obesity crises unless it addresses their psychological underpinnings. With the tools of cognitive therapy, a healthy internal parent voice, and discipline, you can start to do this in your own life. You can develop wisdom, maturity, responsibility and character strength to help you rise to every challenge that life brings you. A fantastic way to practice this, as you know, is through journaling. Keeping up a meal diary and journal allows you to continually check in on how you're doing with your personal goals for health eating and living.

Yes, the knowledge you have gained is like currency. Use it well, invest in your own health, and the returns on your investment will be endless. Bury it away and forget you ever had it, and you'll have squandered a wonderful opportunity to better your quality of life.

Don't ever let yourself be the victim when it comes to your health. Don't let yourself get away with excuses. *You* have the power to change. You, and only you, are responsible for taking care of your body.

But here's the key: it has to be something you *want*. Change doesn't come from following orders or from a feeling of duty. So anytime you reluctantly think to yourself, *I should eat vegetables with my meal* or *I shouldn't eat dessert*, stop and think: *Isn't this something I want for myself? Don't I want to take care of the one body I am given on this earth?* If so, then rephrase those statements: "I *want* to eat vegetables with my meal," and "I *don't want* to eat dessert." If you truly care about your health, then those statements are 100 percent genuine.

It is this shift—from an attitude of reluctant sacrifice to one of willing and joyful nurturance—that is absolutely crucial to success. You must view the changes you're making as life-giving, restorative, and *beautiful*.

It won't always be easy. There will be ups and downs in this path to success. But you mustn't lose heart when the going gets rough. And don't get discouraged when you slip up. Learn from your mistakes. Examine why they happened. Did you unintentionally set yourself up for that midnight binge by starving yourself all day, skipping meals, or exercising for hours on end?

You'll have to be honest with yourself though. Shine a light into the deep recesses of your mind to illuminate any deep-seated, underlying issues you have that are preventing you from succeeding. It might hurt to be so brutally honest with yourself. But if disordered eating habits are stemming from a deeper psychological issue (as they often are), then there's no way to fully conquer them without addressing the underlying reasons for their existence.

Examining all the possible psychological reasons for disordered eating is beyond the scope of this book, but to get you started, here are some questions to ask yourself:

- Am I using eating as a means of comforting myself? Is food something I turn to to relieve loneliness, sadness, shame, or hurt?

  Identify any reasons you might have for emotional eating and choose to confront those head-on rather than using food as a decoy. Put your feelings into words—in a journal or to a friend or therapist—not into food.

- Are my disordered eating habits a means of rebellion?

  Identify who or what you're trying to rebel against. Is it your parents? Societal norms?

- Am I trying to express my autonomy by showing that I can do whatever I want with my body, even if it's detrimental to my health?

  Express your autonomy in a positive and real way. You have every right to assert your individuality. But don't do it in a self-destructive manner.

- Do I feel like I don't have a voice? Or like I'm not seen? Is my disordered eating behavior really a cry for help or attention?

  Find your true voice. Bravely seek out the help you need and deserve.

- Do I overeat to show the world I don't care what people think of me? Is this really just a big "F*** you" to the norms of society?

  This may come from a lack of self-esteem due to a feeling of rejection—a feeling that you don't fit in. Work through the issues that prevent you from loving your true self in all its messiness and even brokenness. Your immeasurable value as a person is inherent: It doesn't come from outside sources; you don't need others' approval to validate it. *Learn to love the imperfect self.*

- Have I been using food restriction as a way to feel in control when my life seems to be spinning out of control?

  What feels out of control in your life? Discern which of those things are in your hands and which are out of your hands. You have control over your college applications; be proactive and do them as best you can. But you don't have control over college admissions decisions. Likewise, you don't have control over your daughter who has run away from home or your husband who has turned to drinking. The only person you have control over is yourself. Focus on establishing those boundaries rather than hiding behind controlling eating patterns.

It might take years, a lifetime even, to address some of these deeper issues. And it will probably hurt to look your monsters square in the eye instead of ignoring or denying their existence. But confronting those wounds and fears head-on is the only way toward healing and progress.

The good news is you don't necessarily need to dole out the big bucks to work through these issues with a psychiatrist. You can practice cognitive therapy on yourself. You know how to do that now, and the best way is through journaling. Ask yourself the hard questions, dig into your past, and find the root of your problems. It will take bravery and honesty, but it will be worth it in the end.

Mastery

In George Leonard's best-selling book, *Mastery: The Keys to Success and Long-Term Fulfillment*, he outlines five steps to mastery.[6] I think they're so spot on that I'd like to conclude by examining these steps in light of our quest for health.

1. *Instruction*: As I said earlier, knowledge empowers you with the tools you need for success. Don't stop with this book. Devote yourself to being a student of the ever-developing science of nutrition.

2. *Practice*: This is perhaps the most difficult concept to employ, but the most important to the development of mastery. It's difficult, because people like mountaintop experiences—the celebration of positive results—but hate the plateaus, the tedious, day-to-day practice. Leonard says, "To love the plateau is to love what is most essential and enduring in your life." It is through practice that a novel experience becomes the intricate rhythm of one's life.

3. *Surrender*: To surrender means to give up, to declare defeat, to become broken. Change occurs once we surrender to the call to wisdom and give ourselves over to the practice of discipline. Abandon your old patterns. Take the plunge. No one can do this for you.

4. *Intentionality*: Visualize your plans, focus on your goals. Live it, be it, know who you are and who you want to become. All of this gives meaning to the mundane.

5. *The Edge*: This is the advantage that you can and *will* have if your passion for excellence is sustained over time. When you know the facts, when you can tolerate tedious repetition, when

you learn to love the plateaus, when you find the joy in the subtlest elements of change, when you surrender to the process, and when you find your ability to sustain passion, you can master any discipline.

I wish you the very best of luck on this journey toward mastery and toward a healthier you. May you have the courage, the motivation, and the discipline to become all that you want to be—all that you deserve to be.

APPENDIX

Just for Laughs: A *South Park* Rendition of the Gluten-Free Craze

"Gluten Free Ebola" Synopsis:

Mr. Mackey is now gluten free, and everyone is annoyed when he won't quit preaching about how great he feels. But after witnessing a disturbing demonstration of what happens to your body when you do eat gluten, South Park becomes the first town in America to go gluten free.[1, 2, 3]

[The Marsh house. The bell rings and Randy answers it.]

Randy:	Yes?
Worker 1:	Hello, sir. We've had word of a possible gluten exposure in your home. May we come in?
Randy:	Gluten expo … Oh not here!
Worker 2:	Can we come in please?
Randy:	Wuh sure! *[Shows them in. They enter and their gluten meters crackle as they go around the house.]*
Sharon:	*[Coming down the stairs]* What's going on? *[One of the workers stops at the kitchen wastebasket and pulls out a pair of tongs. He rifles through the trash can with it and pulls out a Pabst Blue Ribbon can.]*
Randy:	Well, that's just a beer …
Shelly:	Beer is all wheat, Dad!

Randy:	*[To Shelly]* Shuut up. *[To the worker]* Beer is bad for you?
Worker 2:	We're gonna need you to come with us, sir. Don't touch me ...
Worker 1:	We just need you to be in quarantine for a while until everyone figures out what's going on.
Randy:	No! Not Papa John's. *[Shakes his head.]* I don't wanna go to Papa John's! *[Shakes his head more violently.]* You can't make me go to Papa Jooohn's!

[Papa John's, day. It is now Gluten Quarantine Center 1, and Randy's the newest quarantine. Outside are one of the workers and a soldier.]

Randy:	How long do I have to stay here?
Soldier:	Until the USDA gets control of the situation, sir.
Randy:	What am I supposed to eat?
Soldier:	It's okay; there's lots of toppings. Just eat the toppings.

[The soldier and the worker walk away]

A Quarantine:	How'd you get exposed? *[It's a blond man on the floor.]* Bagels? Gravy?
Randy:	Beer. I didn't know it had gluten.
Mr. Garrison:	There's always somethin'. For me, it was the soy sauce. *[His voice grows soft.]* Sneaky, sneaky soy sauce.

[USDA headquarters, day]

Jeff:	We're trying to get a handle on just how much gluten there is out there, but ... it seems impossible to contain.
Tom Vilsack:	And we have no idea how to tell people to protect themselves?
Researcher:	*[Approaches with an open laptop]* We've been running simulations, but they're problematic because they don't relate to our current schematics. Here, look. This is what we've been recommending for the past three years. *[Shown is a food tray with a dish and cup on it. The dish has larger portions for veggies and grains,*

smaller portions for fruits and proteins, and the cup is dairy, off to the side with the smallest portion.] Five basic food groups, not four. We were wrong about that. We now realize, of course, that the largest of these groups we've been recommending is basically poison. [*A skull and crossbones appears over the grains*]. Sir, to combat the gluten, we're trying every possible combination of the four remaining food groups, but so far, no answers.

[*USDA headquarters, day. Everyone is in a rush.*]

Tom Vilsack: It's dinnertime on the East Coast in less than an hour. People are going to die!

Jeff White: Sir! They've got a boy on the hotline who says he might know something.

Tom Vilsack: Who is this?

Cartman: My name isn't important. What matters is that ... the answer is in the pyramid.

Tom Vilsack: The pyramid? That's ancient stuff you're talking about. Are you sure? [*To the floor*] Bring up the pyramid! [*A programmer gets on it. An image comes up on screen, showing four food groups in four layers inside a pyramid. Grains take the bottom, widest layer, followed by fruits and vegetables, meat and dairy, and fats and oils narrowing to a point at the top.*]

Cartman: What, what is it? What is it for?

Tom Vilsack: We built the pyramid a long time ago to illustrate how much people should eat of the four basic food groups.

Programmer: Sir, we abandoned the pyramid when Michelle Obama got involved.

Tom Vilsack: The pyramid doesn't work. We already tried it.

Cartman: It's upside down.

Tom Vilsack: What?

Cartman: Sir, the pyramid is upside down.

Tom Vilsack: Turn the pyramid upside down.

Programmer 2: You can't be serious. That would put butter and fat at the top of the—

Tom Vilsack: Flip the damned food pyramid!

Michael Taylor: This is *not* FDA-approved!

Tom Vilsack: It's dinnertime on the East Coast in ten minutes! Now *do it*! [*The programmers get on it.*]

Programmer 3: Sir, we've got a match.

Programmer 4: Nutrition is stabilizing!

Programmer 5: We've got a well-balanced vaccine, sir! [*Everyone cheers.*]

Tom Vilsack: Get the president on the phone. Tell him ... to have some steak with his butter.

NOTES

Preface

1   R. Lavizzo-Mourey and J. Levi, "What Is the State of Obesity in America?" *The State of Obesity*. Accessed July 19, 2016. http://stateofobesity.org/letter/.

2   M. Fox, "America's Obesity Epidemic Hits a New High," *NBC News*. June 7, 2016. http://www.nbcnews.com/health/health-news/america-s-obesity-epidemic-hits-new-high-n587251.

Chapter 1: A Disordered Eating Society

1   Centers for Disease Control and Prevention (May 18, 2015), http://www.cdc/nchs/fastats/overwt.htm.

2   Ibid.

3   "Eating Disorders 101 Guide: A Summary of Issues, Statistics and Resources," The Renfrew Center Foundation for Eating Disorders (2003).

4   "Eating Disorders Statistics," n.d., http://www.anad.org/get-information/about-eating-disorders/eating-disorders-statistics/.

5   J. Reedy and S. M. Krebs-Smith, "Dietary Sources of Energy, Solid Fats, and Added Sugars among Children and Adolescents in the United States," *Journal of the American Dietetic Association* 110, no. 10 (October 2010), 1477–1484, http://www.ncbi.nlm.nih.gov/pubmed/20869486.

6   "Dietary Guidelines for Americans," US Department of Agriculture (2010), http://www.cnpp.usda.gov/dietaryguidelines.htm.

7   Image from U.S. Department of Agriculture, Past Food Pyramid Materials (June 1, 2011), https://fnic.nal.usda.gov/dietary-guidance/myplate-and-historical-food-pyramid-resources/past-food-pyramid-materials.

8   A. Gustafson-Larson and R. D. Terry, "Weight-Related Behaviors and Concerns of Fourth-Grade Children," *Journal of the American Dietetic Association* 92 (1992): 818–822.

Chapter 2: Dieting: The Gateway Drug

1   Data and Statistics, Centers for Disease Control (September 14, 2015), http://www.cdc.gov/obesity/data/index.html.

2   *Consumer Reports Diet Survey* (April 1, 2007), http://www.wral.com/asset/5oys/2007/05/07/1393071/1178575321_ConsumerReportsDietSurvey.pdf.

3   J. Zaslow, "Girls and Dieting, Then and Now" (September 2009), http://www.wsj.com/articles/SB10001424052970204731804574386822245731710.

4   W. F. Boyce, M. A. King, and J. Roche, "Healthy Living and Healthy Weight in Healthy Settings for Young People in Canada" (2008), http://www.phac-aspc.gc.ca/dca-dea/yic/pdf/youth-jeunes-eng.pdf.

5   L. M. Mellin, C. E. Irwin, and S. Scully, "Disordered Eating Characteristics in Girls: A Survey of Middle Class Children," *Journal of the American Dietetic Association* (1992): 851–53.

6   C. Kurth, D. Krahn, K. Nairn, and A. Drewnowski, "The Severity of Dieting and Bingeing Behaviors in College Women: Interview Validation of Survey Data," *Journal of Psychiatric Research* (1995): 211–225.

7   A. Gustafson-Larson and R. D. Terry, "Weight-Related Behaviors and Concerns of Fourth-Grade Children," *Journal of the American Dietetic Association* 92 (1992): 818–822.

8   H. Dalzell, "Pathological Dieting: Precursor to Eating Disorders," (July 14, 2010), http://www.examiner.com/eating-disorder-in-philadelphia/pathological-dieting-precursor-to-eating-disorders.

9   J. Cogan, J. Smith, and M. Maine, "The Risks of a Quick Fix: A Case against Mandatory Body Mass Index Reporting Laws," *Eating Disorders* 16 (2007): 2–13.

10 D. Neumark-Sztainer, M. Story, P. J. Hannan, C. L. Perry, and L. M. Irving, "Weight-Related Concerns and Behaviors among Overweight and Nonoverweight Adolescents," *Archives of Pediatrics and Adolescent Medicine* 156, no. 2 (2002): 171–178, http://www.medic.Ca/knowthefacts/statistics.shtml.

11 M. Schwartz, L. Vartanian, B. Nosek, and K. Brownell, "The Influence of One's Own Body Weight on Implicit and Explicit Antifat Bias," *Obesity* 14, no. 3 (2006): 440–447.

12 Ibid.

13 G. Gaesser, *Big Fat Lies: The Truth about Your Weight and Your Health* (New York: Fawcett Columbine, 1996).

14 Ibid.

15 War on Obesity (July 4, 2013), http://www.bigfatfacts.com/uncategorized/war-on-obesity/.

16 T. Mann, A. J. Tomiyama, E. Westling, A. M. Lew, B. Samuels, and J. Chatman, "Medicare's Search for Effective Obesity Treatments—Diets Are Not the Answer," *American Psychologist* 62 (2007): 220–233.

17 S. Wolpert, "Dieting Does Not Work," *UCLA Researchers Report* (April 3, 2007), http://newsroom.ucla.edu/portal/ucla/Dieting-Does-Not-Work-UCLA-Researchers-7832.aspx?RelNum=7832.

18 C. Lagorio, "Diet Plan Success Tough to Weigh," *CBS News*, January 3, 2005, http://www.cbsnews.com/2100-204_162-664519.html.

19 "Statistics on Weight Discrimination: A Waste of Talent," n.d., http://www.cswd.org/index.html.

20 E. Stice, R. Cameron, J. Killen, C. Hayward, and C. Taylor, "Naturalistic Weight-Reduction Efforts Prospectively Predict Growth in Relative Weight and Onset of Obesity among Female Adolescents," *Journal of Consulting and Clinical Psychology* (1999): 967–974.

21 C. M. Shisslak, M. Crago, and L. S. Estes, "The Spectrum of Eating Disturbances," *International Journal of Eating Disorders* 18, no. 3 (1995): 209–219.

22 K. Brownell, M. Greenwood, E. Stellar, and E. Shrager, "The Effects of Repeated Cycles of Weight Loss and Regain in Rats," *Physiology & Behavior* 38 (1986): 459–464.

23 A. G. Dulloo and L. Girardier, "Adaptive Changes in Energy Expenditure during Refeeding Following Low Calorie Intake: Evidence for a Specific Metabolic Component Favoring Fat Storage," *American Journal of Clinical Nutrition* 52 (1990): 415–420.

24 C. E. Adams and M. R. Leary, "Promoting Self–Compassionate Attitudes Toward Eating Among Restrictive and Guilty Eaters," *Journal of Social and Clinical Psychology* 26, no. 10 (2007): 1120-144. doi:10.1521/jscp.2007.26.10.1120.

25 P. Boyle, L. Storlien, and R. Keesey, "Increased Efficiency of Food Utilization Following Weight Loss," *Physiology & Behavior* 21 (1978): 261–264.

26 R. Hassin, K. Ochsner, and Y. Trope, "Self-Control in Society, Mind, and Brain," *Oxford University Press* (2010): 379–379, http://180degreehealth.com/2011/11/restrained-eating-and-obesity.

27 T. Tucker, *The Great Starvation Experiment: Ancel Keys and the Men Who Starved for Science* (Minneapolis: University of Minnesota Press, 2007).

28 J. K. Rowling, *Harry Potter and the Goblet of Fire* (New York: Levine Scholastic, 2000).

29 "The Psychology of Dieting," The National Center for Eating Disorders, http://www.eating-disorder.org.uk/psychology-of-dieting.html.

30 A. Keys, *The Biology of Human Starvation* (Minneapolis: University of Minnesota Press, 1950).

Chapter 3: Diets Gone Wild

1 M. Spearing, "Eating Disorders: Facts about Eating Disorders and the Search for Solutions," PsycEXTRA Dataset, n.d., www.carf.org/WorkArea/DownloadAsset.aspx?id=22448.

2 "Eating Disorders Statistics," National Association of Anorexia and Associated Disorders, n.d., http://www.anad.org/get-information/about-eating-disorders/eating-disorders-statistics/.

3 "Dispelling the Shame and Secrecy of Eating Disorders" (January 31, 2011), http://mommiesmagazine.com/10405/dispelling-shame-secrecy-eating/.

4 D. J. Carlat and C. A. Camargo, "Review of Bulimia Nervosa in Males," *American Journal of Psychiatry* 148, no. 7 (July 1991): 831–43.

5 D. J. Carlat, C. A. Camargo Jr., and M. D. Herzog, "Eating Disorders in Males: A Report on 135 patients," *American Journal of Psychiatry* 154, no. 8 (August 1997): 1127–1132.

6 South Carolina Department of Mental Health, n.d., http://www.state.sc.us/dmh/anorexia/statistics.htm.

7 The Alliance for Eating Disorders Awareness, https://www.ndsu.edu/fileadmin/counseling/Eating_Disorder_Statistics.pdf.

8 E. Mash, *Assessment of Childhood Disorders*, 3rd ed. (New York: Guilford Press, 1997).

9 E. Cooney, (2010, November 29). "Genes, Puberty, and Weight in Women," *Boston Globe*, November 29, 2010, http://www.boston.com/lifestyle/family/articles/2010/11/29/genes_puberty_and_weight_in_women/.

10 Ibid.

11 L. Smolak, *Next Door Neighbors Puppet Guidebook*, National Eating Disorders Association (1996).

12 *Mean Girls*, M. Waters (Director), T. Fey (Screenwriter), Motion picture, Paramount (2004).

13 M. Levine, "Prevention of Eating Problems with Elementary Children," *USA Today*, July 1998.

14 L. Smolak and M. Levine, "Body Image, Disordered Eating, and Eating Disorders," *The Wiley Handbook of Eating Disorders Smolak / The Wiley Handbook of Eating Disorders* (2015): 1–10.

15 N. Digate Muth, "What Are the Guidelines for Percentage of Body Fat Loss?" American Council on Exercise (December 2, 2009), http://www.acefitness.org/acefit/healthy-living-article/60/112/what-are-the-guidelines-for-percentage-of/.

16 R. L. Levine, "The Medical Minute: Eating Disorders Affect Entire Body," *Penn State Live* (February 25, 2004), http://live.psu.edu/story/5753.

17 L. Smolak, *Next Door Neighbors Puppet Guidebook*, National Eating Disorders Association (1996).

18 R. Rettner, "Girls' Food Choices at Age 9 May Predict Future Eating Disorders," *Fox News*, May 31, 2012, http://www.foxnews.com/health/2012/05/31/girls-food-choices-at-age-may-predict-future-eating-disorders/.

19 "Practice Guidelines for Eating Disorders," *American Journal of Psychiatry* 150, no. 2 (1993): 212–228.

20 "Eating Disorders 101 Guide: A Summary of Issues, Statistics, and Resources," *The Renfrew Center Foundation for Eating Disorders* (2002), http://www.renfrew.org.

21 Ibid.

22 *Diagnostic and Statistical Manual of Mental Disorders: DSM-IV-TR*, 4th ed. (Washington, DC: American Psychiatric Association, 2000).

23 C. Coffey, *Pediatric Neuropsychiatry* (Philadelphia, PA: Lippincott Williams & Wilkins, 2006): 309–312.

24 W. Kaye, "Neurobiology of Anorexia and Bulimia Nervosa," *Physiology and Behavior* (November 29, 2007), http://www2.massgeneral.org/harriscenter/about_an.asp.

25 U. F. Bailer and W. H. Kaye, "A Review of Neuropeptide and Neuroendocrine Dysregulation in Anorexia and Bulimia Nervosa," *Current Drug Targets—CNS and Neurological Disorders* 2 (2003): 53–59.

26 D. Katzman, "Medical Complications in Adolescents with Anorexia Nervosa: A Review of the literature," *International Journal of Eating Disorders* 37 (2005): 552–559.

27 R. L. Pyle, J. E. Mitchell, and E. D. Eckert, "Bulimia: A Report of 34 Cases," *Journal of Clinical Psychiatry*, 42 (1981): 60–64.

28 A. H. Crisp, "The Possible Significance of Some Behavioral Correlates of Weight and Carbohydrate Intake," *Journal of Psychosomatic Research* 11, no. 1 (June 1967): 117–131.

29 P. Dally and J. Gomez, *Anorexia Nervosa* (London: William Heinemann, 1979).

30 M. Apfelbaum, J. Bostsarron, and D. Lacatis, "Effect of Caloric Restriction and Excessive Caloric Intake on Energy Expenditure," *American Journal of Clinical Nutrition* 24, no. 12 (December 1971): 1405–9.

31 G. W. Bo-Linn, C. A. Santa Ana, S. G. Morawski, and J. S. Fordtran, "Purging and Calorie Absorption in Bulimic Patients and Normal Women," *Annals of Internal Medicine* 99 (1983): 14–27.

32 G. W. Bo-Linn, C. A. Santa Ana, S. G. Morawski, and J. S. Fordtran, "Purging and Calorie Absorption in Bulimic Patients and Normal Women," *Annals of Internal Medicine* 99 (1983): 14–27.

33 J. Garrow, *Energy Balance and Obesity in Man* (New York: Elsevier, 1974).

34 "Bulimia Nervosa," n.d., http://www.mayoclinic.org/diseases-conditions/bulimia/basics/complications/con-20033050.

35 J. M. Rushing, L. E. Jones, and C. P. Carney, (2003). "Bulimia Nervosa: A Primary Care Review Primary Care Companion," *Journal of Clinical Psychiatry* 5, no. 5 (2003): 217–224.

36 "Eating Disorders Statistics," n.d., *Anorexia Nervosa & Related Eating Disorders*, https://www.anred.com/stats.html.

37 Roland L. Weinsier, G. Hunter, R. A. Desmond, N. M. Byrne, P. A. Zuckerman, B. E. Darnell, "Free-Living Activity Energy Expenditure in Women Successful and Unsuccessful at Maintaining a Normal Body Weight," *Am J Clin Nutrition* 75, no. 3 (2002): 499–504.

38 Manfred J. Muller, Anja Bosy-Westphal, and Steven B. Heymsfield, "Is There Evidence for a Set Point that Regulates Human Body Weight?" *Med Rep* 2, no. 59 (2010).

39 M. D. Hensrud, "Is Too Little Sleep a Cause of Weight Gain?" Mayo Clinic (2015), accessed May 26, 2016, http://www.mayoclinic.com/health/sleep-and-weight-gain/AN02178.

40 E. S. Epel, B. McEwen, T. Seeman, K. Matthews, G. Castellazzo, K. D. Brownell, J Bell, J.R. Ickovics, "Stress and Body Shape: Stress-Induced Cortisol Secretion Is Consistently Greater among Women with Central Fat," *Psychosomatic Medicine* 62 (2000): 623–632.

41 T. D. Wade, A. Keski-Rahkonen, and J. Hudson, "Epidemiology of Eating Disorders," *Textbook in Psychiatric Epidemiology*, 3rd ed., eds. M. Tsuang and M. Tohen (New York: Wiley, 2011), 343–360.

42 "Eating Disorder Statistics and Research," n.d., http://www.eatingdisorderhope.com/information/statistics-studies#Prevalence-of-eating-disorders-among-athletes.

43 "Disordered Eating in Student-Athletes: Understanding the Basics and What We Can Do about It," National Collegiate Athletic Association (2014), http://www.ncaa.org/health-and-safety/nutrition-and-performance/disordered-eating-student-athletes-understanding-basics.

44 "Eating Disorder Statistics and Research," n.d., http://www.eatingdisorderhope.com/information/statistics-studies#Prevalence-of-eating-disorders-among-athletes.

45 R. Ringham, K. Klump, W. Kaye, D. Stone, S. Libman, S Stowe, and M. Marcus, "Eating Disorder Symptomatology among Ballet Dancers," *Int J Eat Disord* 39 (2006): 503–508.

46 "Weight 'Cutting' Waning among College Wrestlers," *Eating Disorders Review* 14, no. 5 (2003), http://eatingdisordersreview.com/nl/nl_edr_14_5_7.html.

47 "Nutrition and Athletic Performance," *Medicine & Science in Sports & Exercise* 41 no. 3 (2009): 709–731.

48 S. John, "I'm Not Fat, Says Ballerina Faulted for 'Too Many Sugarplums,'" *Today News* (2010), http://www.today.com/id/40639920/ns/today-today_news/t/im-not-fat-says-ballerina-faulted-too-many-sugarplums/#.V0c49ucrK00.

49 T. Benn and D. Walters, "Between Scylla and Charybdis: Nutritional Education Versus Body Culture and the Ballet Aesthetic: The Effects on the Lives of Female Dancers," *Research in Dance Education* 2, no. 2 (2001): 139–154.

50 E. L. Lowenkopf and L. M. Vincent, "The Student Ballet Dancer and Anorexia," *Hillside Journal of Clinical Psychiatry* 4 (1982): 53–64.

51 D. Ice Grange, J. Tibbs, and T. D. Noakes, "Implications of Anorexia Nervosa in a Ballet School," *Int J Eat Disord* 15 (1994): 369–37.

52 E. L. Lowenkopf and L. M. Vincent, "The Student Ballet Dancer and Anorexia," *Hillside Journal of Clinical Psychiatry* 4 (1982): 53–64.

53 "Nutrition and Athletic Performance," *Medicine & Science in Sports & Exercise* 41, no. 3 (2009): 709–731.

Chapter 4: How Our Bodies Use Food

1 J. Weisenberger, "Understanding Calories," n.d., http://www.innerbody.com/nutrition/understanding-calories.

2 "All Calories Are Not Created Equal," n.d., http://www.lazaruslabs.com/all-calories-are-not-created-equal.

3 D. Paddon-Jones and E. Westman, "Protein, Weight Management, and Satiety," *The American Journal of Clinical Nutrition* 87 (2008).

4 Roland L. Weinsier, G. Hunter, R. Desmond, N. Byrne, P. Zuckerman, and B. Darnell, "Free-Living Activity Energy Expenditure in Women Successful and Unsuccessful at Maintaining a Normal Body Weight," *American Journal of Clinical Nutrition* 75, no. 3 (March 2002): 499–504.

5 Eastman, C. J., and M. Li. "The Changing Epidemiology of Iodine Deficiency : Article ..." April 3, 2012. Accessed September 3, 2016. http://www.nature.com/nrendo/journal/v8/n7/full/nrendo.2012.43.html.

6 M. J. Muller, A. Bosy-Westphal, and S. Heymsfield, "Is There Evidence for a Set Point that Regulates Human Body Weight?" *Journal of Medical Case Reports* (2010).

7 J. Duvauchelle, "The Effects of Low Protein Intake" (January 27, 2015), http://www.livestrong.com/article/214483-the-effects-of-low-protein-intake/.

8 N. J. Rothwell and M. J. Stock, "Influence of Carbohydrate and Fat Intake on Diet-Induced Thermogenesis and Brown Fat Activity in Rats Fed Low Protein Diets," *The Journal of Nutrition* 117, no. 10 (1987): 1721–1726.

9 "Amino Acids," n.d., http://www.biology.arizona.edu/biochemistry/problem_sets/aa/aa.html.

10 H. Nemets, B. Nemets, A. Apter, Z. Bracha, and R. H. Belmaker, "Omega-3 Treatment of Childhood Depression: A Controlled, Double-Blind Pilot Study," *American Journal of Psychiatry* 163, no. 6 (2006): 1098–1100.

11 V. Anand, "Myths about Lowering Cholesterol" (March 29, 2012), http://www.onlymyhealth.com/myths-about-lowering-cholesterol-1324036783.

12 J. Pottala, K. Yaffe, J. Robinson, M. Espeland, R. Wallace, and W. Harris, "Higher RBC EPA DHA Corresponds with Larger Total Brain and Hippocampal Volumes: WHIMS-MRI Study," *Neurology* (2014): 435–442.

13 M. Hyman, *The UltraMind Solution* (New York, NY: Simon and Schuster/Scribner, 2009).

14 W. P. Castelli, "Concerning the Possibility of a Nut ..." *Archives of Internal Medicine* 152, no. 7 (July 1992): 1371–2.

15 N. Stoyanova, "Mediterranean Diet May Be the Secret to Longevity" (February 4, 2008), http://www.naturalnews.com/022583_diet_mediterranean_health.html.

16 E. Huff, "Dr. George V. Mann | HealthWars.co.," (January 22, 2012), http://healthwars.co/tag/dr-george-v-mann/.

17 A. P. Simopoulos, "The Importance of the Omega-6/Omega-3 Fatty Acid Ratio in Cardiovascular Disease and Other Chronic Diseases," *Experimental Biology and Medicine* 223, no. 6 (2008): 674–88.

18 C. Kresser, "How Too Much Omega-6 and Not Enough Omega-3 Is Making Us Sick" (May 8, 2010), http://chriskresser.com/how-too-much-omega-6-and-not-enough-omega-3-is-making-us-sick/.

19 "Simple Answers for Healthier Families, n.d., http://wellnessmama.com.

20 "Fatty Acid Imbalance Increases the Risk of Depression and Heart Disease" (April 23, 2007), http://www.doctorshealthpress.com/anti-aging/arthritis/an-imbalance-of-fatty-acids-could-increase-your-risk-of-depression-and-heart-disease.

21 L. Robinson, J. Segal, and R. Segal, "Choosing Healthy Fats: Good Fats, Bad Fats, and the Power of Omega-3s" (December 2015), http://www.helpguide.org/articles/healthy-eating/choosing-healthy-fats.htm.

22 "Healing Foods Pyramid," n.d., http://www.med.umich.edu/umim/food-pyramid/fats.html.

23 Y. Elkaim, "The Shocking Truth about Sunflower Oil" (January 3, 2014), http://health.usnews.com/health-news/blogs/eat-run/2014/01/03/the-shocking-truth-about-sunflower-oil.

24 A. P. Simopoulos, "The Importance of the Omega-6/Omega-3 Fatty Acid Ratio in Cardiovascular Disease and Other Chronic Diseases," *Experimental Biology and Medicine* 223, no. 6 (2008): 674–88.

25 K. Hartel, "Which Cooking Oil Is the Best One for You?" n.d., http://www.fitday.com/fitness-articles/nutrition/which-cooking-oil-is-the-best-one-for-you.html.

26 J. Mercola, "What Oil Should You Be Cooking with, and Which Should You Avoid?" (October 15, 2003), http://articles.mercola.com/sites/articles/archive/2003/10/15/cooking-oil.aspx.

27 Ibid.

28 R. Andrews, "All about Lectins: Here's What You Need to Know" (August 10, 2009), http://www.precisionnutrition.com/all-about-lectins.

29 "Lectins, Phytates and Gluten Free Diet—Only Gluten Free Recipes" (September 12, 2014), http://onlyglutenfreerecipes.com/lectins-phytates-and-gluten-free-diet/.

30 M. Edwards, "How Gluten and Candida Cause Leaky Gut," *Natural News* (May 12, 2015), http://www.naturalnews.com/049674_gluten_intolerance_candida_albicans_leaky_gut.html.

31 B. T. Cooper, G. K. Holmes, and W. T. Cooke, "Coeliac Disease and Immunological Disorders," *British Medical Journal* 1, no. 6112 (1978): 537–539, doi:10.1136/bmj.1.6112.537.

32 "Gluten May Cause Depression in People with Non-Celiac Gluten Sensitivity," Celiac Disease Foundation (July 17, 2014), https://celiac.org/blog/2014/07/gluten-may-cause-depression-people-non-celiac-gluten-sensitivity/.

33 S. Boyles, "Gluten Intolerance Linked to Schizophrenia," WebMD (February 20, 2004), http://www.webmd.com/schizophrenia/news/20040219/gluten-intolerance-linked-to-schizophrenia.

34 K. Rostami, E. A. Steegers, W. Y. Wong, D. D. Braat, and R. P. Steegers-Theunissen, "Coeliac Disease and Reproductive Disorders: A Neglected Association," *Eur J Obstet Gynecol Reprod Biol* 96, no. 2 (2001): 146–9.

35 N. M. Lau, P. H. Green, A. K. Taylor, D. Hellberg, M. Ajamian, C. Z. Tan, and A. Alaedini, "Markers of Celiac Disease and Gluten Sensitivity

in Children with Autism," PLoS ONE, 8, no. 6 (2013), doi:10.1371/journal.pone.0066155.

36 F. L. Soares, R. D. Matoso, L. G. Teixeira, Z. Menezes, S. S. Pereira, A. C. Alves, and J. I. Alvarez-Leite, "Gluten-Free Diet Reduces Adiposity, Inflammation, and Insulin Resistance Associated with the Induction of PPAR-alpha and PPAR-gamma Expression," *The Journal of Nutritional Biochemistry* 24, no. 6 (2013): 1105–1111, doi:10.1016/j.jnutbio.2012.08.009.

37 "Why Is Wheat Gluten Disorder on the Rise," (June 23, 2009), Mercola.com, http://articles.mercola.com/sites/articles/archive/2009/07/23/why-is-wheat-gluten-disorder-on-the-rise.aspx.

38 "Gluten Allergy Now Four Times More Common Than in the 1950s," *WorldHealth.net* (July 7, 2009), http://www.worldhealth.net/news/gluten_allergy_now_four_times_more_commo/.

39 "Why Is Wheat Gluten Disorder on the Rise," Mercola.com (June 23, 2009), http://articles.mercola.com/sites/articles/archive/2009/07/23/why-is-wheat-gluten-disorder-on-the-rise.aspx.

40 Ibid.

41 R. Andrews, "All about Lectins: Here's What You Need to Know" (August 10, 2009), http://www.precisionnutrition.com/all-about-lectins.

42 M. Ravensthorpe, "Three Mucilaginous Foods that Make Great Natural Laxatives" (July 18, 2014), http://www.naturalnews.com/046045_natural_laxatives_foods_okra.html.

Chapter 5: The Glycemic Index

1 A. M. Harvey, R. J. Johns, V. A. McKusick, A. H. Owens Jr., and R. S. Ross, The Principles and Practice of Internal Medicine, 20th ed. (New York: Appleton Century Crofts, 1980).

2 L. W. David and V. Marks, *Scientific Foundations of Biochemistry in Clinical Practice*, Butterworth-Heinemann, (September 1994).

3 *Statistics about Diabetes: National Diabetes Statistics Report* (June 10, 2014).

4 R. C. Rabin, "Diabetes on the Rise among Teenagers," May 21, 2012, http://well.blogs.nytimes.com/2012/05/21/diabetes-on-the-rise-among-teenagers/.

5 R. Brodsky, "Type 2 Diabetes and the Glycemic Index," *Diabetes Daily Post* (May 24, 2012), http://diabetesdailypost.com/type-2-diabetes-and-the-glycemic-index/.

6 "Glycemic Index and Glycemic Load for 100 Foods," *Harvard Health* (August 27, 2015), http://www.health.harvard.edu/healthy-eating/glycemic_index_and_glycemic_load_for_100_foods.

7   "Fiber," *The Nutrition Source*, Harvard T. H. Chan School of Public Health, n.d., http://www.hsph.harvard.edu/nutritionsource/carbohydrates/fiber/.

8   A. Guyton and J. Hall, *Textbook of Medical Physiology*, 10th ed. (Philadelphia: WB Saunders, 2000), 936.

9   D. S. Ludwig, J. A. Majzoub, A. Al-Zahrani, G. E. Dallal, I. Blanco, and S. B. Roberts, "High Glycemic Index Foods, Overeating, and Obesity," *Pediatrics* 103 (1999): 261–266.

10   N. Wood, "Wednesday Weight: Week 3" (November 12, 2014), http://www.mylusciouslife.com/wednesday-weight-week-3/.

11   "High and Low Glycemic Index," n.d., http://www.thesnowfairy.com/high-and-low-glycemic-index/.

12   "Healthy Diet: Is Glycemic Index the Key?" *Harvard Health*, n.d., http://www.health.harvard.edu/staying-healthy/healthy-diet-is-glycemic-index-the-key.

13   "Blood Glucose Levels," n.d., http://www.diabetesinc.net/diabetic-level-chart/.

14   R. Langreth and D. Stanford, "Fatty Foods Addictive as Cocaine in Growing Body of Science" (November 1, 2011), http://www.bloomberg.com/news/articles/2011-11-02/fatty-foods-addictive-as-cocaine-in-growing-body-of-science.

15   P. Johnson and P. J. Kenny, "Dopamine D2 Receptors in Addiction-like Reward Dysfunction and Compulsive Eating in Obese Rats," *Nature Neuroscience* 13, no. 50 (2010): 635–4.

16   R. Langreth and D. Stanford, "Fatty Foods Addictive as Cocaine in Growing Body of Science" (November 1, 2011), http://www.bloomberg.com/news/articles/2011-11-02/fatty-foods-addictive-as-cocaine-in-growing-body-of-science.

17   J. Nettleton, P. Lutsey, Y. Wang, J. Lima, E. Michos, and D. Jacobs, "Diet Soda Intake and Risk of Incident Metabolic Syndrome and Type 2 Diabetes in the Multi-Ethnic Study of Atherosclerosis (MESA)," *Diabetes Care* (2009): 688–694.

18   D. DeNoon and Mathus C Grayson, "Drink More Diet Soda, Gain More Weight?" *WebMD: Health News* (June 13, 2005), http://www.webmd.com/diet/20050613/drink-more-diet-soda-gain-more-weight.

Chapter 6: The X-Factor: Xamining Xtreme Xercise

1   "Home—Pure Barre," n.d., http://purebarre.com/.

2   "US Fitness Center / Health Club Revenue 2000–2014 | Statistic," n.d., http://www.statista.com/statistics/236120/us-fitness-center-revenue/.

3   T. Church, C. Earnest, J. Skinner, and S. Blair, "Effects of Different Doses of Physical Activity on Cardiorespiratory Fitness among Sedentary, Overweight or Obese Postmenopausal Women with Elevated Blood Pressure," *JAMA* 19 (2007): 2081–2091.

4   E. John, "Why Exercise Won't Make You Thin," *Observer* (September 18, 2010), http://www.theguardian.com/lifeandstyle/2010/sep/19/exercise-dieting-public-health.

5   G. Reynolds, "Dieting Versus Exercise for Weight Loss," August 1, 2012, http://well.blogs.nytimes.com/2012/08/01/dieting-vs-exercise-for-weight-loss/?_r=0.

6   Ibid.

7   "The Benefits of Exercise," n.d., www2.gsu.edu/~wwwfit/benefits.html.

8   P. Björntorp, "Body Fat Distribution, Insulin Resistance, and Metabolic Diseases," *Nutrition* 13 (1997): 795–803.

9   P. Bjorntorp, "Do Stress Reactions Cause Abdominal Obesity and Comorbidities?" *Obesity Reviews* 2 (2001): 73–86.

10   Ibid.

11   E. John, "Why Exercise Won't Make You Thin," *Observer*, September 18, 2010, http://www.theguardian.com/lifeandstyle/2010/sep/19/exercise-dieting-public-health.

12   J. Mayer and H. E. Rose, "Activity, Calorie Intake, Fat Storage, and the Energy Balance of Infants," *Pediatrics* 41 (1968): 18–29.

13   G. Taubes, "The Scientist and the Stairmaster: Why Most of Us Believe Exercise Makes Us Thinner … and Why We're Wrong," *NYMag.com*, September 24, 2007, http://nymag.com/news/sports/38001/index1.html.

14   P. Björntorp, "Body Fat Distribution, Insulin Resistance, and Metabolic Diseases," *Nutrition* 13 (1997): 795–803.

15   P. Bjorntorp, "Do Stress Reactions Cause Abdominal Obesity and Comorbidities?" *Obesity Reviews* 2 (2001): 73–86.

16   J. Cloud, "Why Exercise Won't Make You Thin," *Time* (August 9, 2009), http://content.time.com/time/magazine/article/0,9171,1914974,00.html.

17   R. Benaroch, Ed., "How Regular Exercise Benefits Teens" (April 11, 2015), http://teens.webmd.com/benefits-of-exercise.

18   "The Benefits of Exercise," n.d., www2.gsu.edu/~wwwfit/benefits.html.

19   P. Björntorp, "Body Fat Distribution, Insulin Resistance, and Metabolic Diseases," *Nutrition* 13 (1997): 795–803.

20   *Legally Blonde*, Rober Leketic (Director), Reese Witherspoon, Luke Wilson, and Selma Blair (Performers), MGM Home Entertainment (2001).

21   P. Björntorp, "Body Fat Distribution, Insulin Resistance, and Metabolic Diseases," *Nutrition* 13 (1997): 795–803.

22 A. Hills, N. King, and N. Byrne, Eds., "Chidren, Obesity, and Exercise: Prevention, Treatment and Management of Childhood and Adolescent Obesity," *International Studies in Physical Education and Youth Sport* 8 (2007): 97–98.

23 J. Mayer, "Inactivity as a Major Factor in Adolescent Obesity," *Annals of the New York Academy of Sciences* (n.d.): 502–506.

24 G. Taubes, *Good Calories, Bad Calories: Challenging the Conventional Wisdom on Diet, Weight Control, and Disease* (New York: Knopf, 2007).

Chapter 7: The Skinny on How to Stay Lean

1 Image from: United States Department of Agriculture, https://commons. wikimedia.org/wiki/File:20111110-OC-AMW-0012_-_Flickr_-_ USDAgov.jpg.

2 "Groups, Pyramids, Labels and Plates: The Evolution of Nutritional Guidelines" (March 6, 2014), http://blog.cambro.com/2014/03/06/groups-pyramids-labels-and-plates-the-evolution-of-nutritional-guidelines/.

3 M. Luckie, "The History of the Food Pyramid" (January 31, 2011), http:// www.washingtonpost.com/wp-srv/special/health/food-pyramid/.

4 Image from United States Department of Agriculture, retrieved from ChooseMyPlate.gov.

5 "The Eating Plan to Burn Fat and Lose Weight," n.d., http://www. menshealth.com/weight-loss/burn-fat-lose-weight.

6 F. F. Samaha, N. Iqbal, P. Seshadri, K.L. Chicano, D.A. Daily, J. Mcgrory, T. Williams, M. Williams, E. J. Gracely, J. Edward and L. Stern, "A Low-Carbohydrate as Compared with a Low-Fat Diet in Severe Obesity," *New England Journal of Medicine* 348 (2003): 2074–81.

7 C. D. Gardner, A. Kiazand, S. Alhassan, et al., "Comparison of the Atkins, Zone, Ornish, and LEARN Diets, the A-Z Weight Loss Study: A Randomized Trial," *Journal of the American Medical Association* (2007): 297, 969–77.

8 J. Nordmann, A. Nordmann, M. Briel, U. Keller, et al., "Effects of Low-Carbohydrate Vs. Low-Fat Diets on Weight Loss and Cardiovascular Risk Factors: A Meta-Analysis of Randomized Controlled Trials," *Archives of Internal Medicine* 166 (2006): 285–293.

9 "Low-Fat Diets Don't Deliver on Heart Health | Atkins," n.d., https:// www.atkins.com/how-it-works/library/articles/low-fat-diets-dont-deliver-on-heart-health.

10 K. Zeratsky, "Does Eating a Healthy Breakfast Help Control Weight?" *Mayo Clinic*, n.d., http://www.mayoclinic.org/healthy-lifestyle/weight-loss/expert-answers/food-and-nutrition/faq-20058449.

Chapter 8: Miracle Foods or Poison?

1   M. Pollan, The Omnivore's Dilemma: A Natural History of Four Meals (New York: Penguin Press, 2006).

2   M. Pollan, *In Defense of Food: An Eater's Manifesto* (New York: Penguin Press, 2008).

3   USDA ERS—Corn. (May 16, 2013), http://www.ers.usda.gov/topics/crops/corn.aspx.

4   M. Pollan, *The Omnivore's Dilemma: A Natural History of Four Meals* (New York: Penguin Press, 2006).

5   M. Pollan, *In Defense of Food: An Eater's Manifesto* (New York: Penguin Press, 2008).

6   K. Daniel, *The Whole Soy Story: The Dark Side of America's Favorite Health Food* (Washington, DC: New Trends Publishing, 2005).

7   Dean Houghton, "Healthful Harvest," *The Furrow* (2000): 10–13.

8   K. Daniel, *The Whole Soy Story: The Dark Side of America's Favorite Health Food* (Washington, DC: New Trends Publishing, 2005).

9   S. Fallon, "The Dangers of Polyunsaturated Vegetable Oils (January 1, 2013), http://healingnaturallybybee.com/the-dangers-of-polyunsaturated-vegetable-oils/. (emphasis added).

10 "Simple Answers for Healthier Families," n.d., http://wellnessmama.com.

11 Ibid.

12 "Margarine Intake and Subsequent Coronary Heart Disease in Men," *Epidemiology* (n.d.), http://journals.lww.com/epidem/Fulltext/1997/03000/Margarine_Intake_and_Subsequent_Coronary_Heart.8.aspx.

13 S. Fallon, "The Dangers of Polyunsaturated Vegetable Oils" (January 1, 2013), http://healingnaturallybybee.com/the-dangers-of-polyunsaturated-vegetable-oils/. (emphasis added).

14 W. Dufty, "Refined Sugar—The Sweetest Poison of All," Global Healing Center (n.d.), http://www.globalhealingcenter.com/sugar-problem/refined-sugar-the-sweetest-poison-of-all.

15 Ibid.

Chapter 9: Superfoods 101

1   R. Bloom, "92% of US Population Have Vitamin Deficiency. Are You One of Them?" The Biostation (February 3, 2014), http://thebiostation.com/resource-center/wellness/92-of-u-s-population-have-vitamin-deficiency-are-you-one-of-them/.

2   "Diet Quality of American School-Age Children by School Lunch Participation Status," Data from the National Health and Nutrition Examination Survey, 1999–2004, Report No. CN-08-NH.

3   M. Murray and J. Pizzorno, *The Encyclopedia of Healing Foods* (New York: Atria Books, 2005).

4   E. Magee, "The Super-Veggies: Cruciferous Vegetables" (April 19, 2007), http://www.webmd.com/food-recipes/super-veggies-cruciferous-vegetables.

5   O. Bond, "Does Ginger Burn Fat?" (May 22, 2015), http://www.livestrong.com/article/440604-does-ginger-burn-fat/.

6   J.F. Stevens, "Vitamin C Detoxifies Oxidized Fat," http://lpi.oregonstate.edu/ss05/oxidizedfat.html.

7   Ibid.

8   T. Walters, *Clean Food: A Seasonal Guide to Eating Close to the Source, with More Than 200 Recipes for a Healthy and Sustainable You* (New York, NY: Sterling, 2009).

9   E. Ward, "Spices and Herbs: Health Benefits and Adding Spices to Foods" (August 5, 2010), http://www.webmd.com/food-recipes/features/spices-and-herbs-health-benefits.

10   M. Hyman, *The UltraMind Solution* (New York, NY: Simon and Schuster/Scribner, 2009).

11   Ibid.

12   "Pecan Superfood Health Benefits and History," *Superfood List* (January 22, 2013), http://superfoodlists.com/pecan-superfood/.

13   "Fats and Cholesterol," Harvard T. H. Chan School of Public Health (n.d.), http://www.hsph.harvard.edu/nutritionsource/what-should-you-eat/fats-and-cholesterol/.

14   "Seafood Health Benefits and Risks," Harvard T. H. Chan School of Public Health (n.d.), http://chge.med.harvard.edu/topic/seafood-health-benefits-risks.

15   "Simple Answers for Healthier Families," *Wellness Mama* (n.d.), http://wellnessmama.com.

16   "Amino Acids" (n.d.), http://www.biology.arizona.edu/biochemistry/problem_sets/aa/aa.html.

17   "Seafood Health Benefits and Risks," Harvard T. H. Chan School of Public Health (n.d.), http://chge.med.harvard.edu/topic/seafood-health-benefits-risks.

18   B. Hornick and E. Yarnell, "Health Benefits of Meat, Poultry, and Fish" (April 16, 2006), http://recipes.howstuffworks.com/fresh-ideas/healthy-dinners/health-benefits-of-meat-poultry-and-fish-gal.html.

19 T. St. John, "A List of Fat-Soluble Vitamins" (January 28, 2015), http://www.livestrong.com/article/282513-a-list-of-fat-soluble-vitamins/.

20 M. Adams, "Dietary Fat Is Necessary for Absorption of Vitamins, Nutrients, and Phytochemicals from Fruits and Vegetables" (July 28, 2004), http://www.naturalnews.com/001545_dietary_fat_good_fats.html.

21 K. Forrest and W. Stuhldreher, "Prevalence and Correlates of Vitamin D Deficiency in US Adults," *Nutrition Research* (2011): 48–54.

22 "Microbiome: Your Body Houses 10x More Bacteria than Cells," http://discovermagazine.com/galleries/zen-photo/m/microbiome.

23 E. Magee, "Yogurt Benefits, Health and Nutrition Facts, and More" (2007), http://www.webmd.com/diet/features/benefits-of-yogurt.

24 J. Rubin, *The Maker's Diet* (Lake Mary, FL: Siloam, 2004).

Chapter 10: Cognitive Therapy

1 "Behavior," Science News 136, no. 23 (1989): 365–365, http://www.jstor.org.ezp-prod1.hul.harvard.edu/stable/3973770.

2 B. A. Alford and A. T. Beck, *The Integrative Power of Cognitive Therapy* (New York: Guilford Press, 1997).

3 J. Holmes, "All You Need Is Cognitive Behaviour Therapy?" *British Medical Journal* 324, no. 7332 (2002): 288–290, http://www.jstor.org.ezp-prod1.hul.harvard.edu/stable/25227348.

4 Barbara Allison, "Parent-Adolescent Conflict in Early Adolescence," *Journal of Family and Consumer Sciences* 2, no. 17 (1998).

5 Plato and I. A. Richards, *Plato's Republic* (Cambridge: Cambridge University Press, 1996).

6 C. Natali, *Aristotle: Nicomachean Ethics* (Oxford: Oxford University Press, 2009).

7 Ibid.

8 C. Natali, *Aristotle: Nicomachean Ethics*, Book 2 (Oxford: Oxford University Press, 2009).

Chapter 12: Final Tips for Success

1 "A Calorie Is Not a Calorie," Pacific Health Laboratories (December 20, 2012), http://home.trainingpeaks.com/blog/article/a-calorie-is-not-a-calorie.

2 R. Myers and M. Mccaleb, "Feeding: Satiety Signal from Intestine Triggers Brain's Noradrenergic Mechanism," *Science* (1980): 1035–1037.

3   "Science Confirms Diet Tactic: Eat Slow, Eat Less" (November 16, 2006), http://www.livescience.com/humanbiology/061115_eating_slow.html.

4   "A Calorie Is Not a Calorie" Pacific Health Laboratories (December 20, 2012), http://home.trainingpeaks.com/blog/article/a-calorie-is-not-a-calorie.

5   M. Healy, "Nighttime Fasting May Foster Weight Loss" (May 18, 2012), http://articles.latimes.com/2012/may/18/science/la-sci-fasting-diet-20120518.

6   G. Leonard, *Mastery: The Keys to Success and Long-Term Fulfillment* (New York, NY: Penguin Books USA Inc., 1992).

Appendix: Just for Laughs—A South Park Rendition of the Gluten-Free Craze

1   T. Parker and M. Stone, "Gluten Free Ebola," Television series episode (October 1, 2014), in *South Park*, Comedy Central.

2   *Wikipedia*, s.v. "Gluten Free Ebola," Accessed May 25, 2016. https://en.wikipedia.org/wiki/Gluten_Free_Ebola.

3   *Wikia*, "Gluten Free Ebola," http://southpark.wikia.com/wiki/Gluten_Free_Ebola#cite_note-0.

ABOUT THE AUTHORS

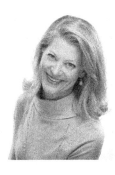

Heidi Wohlrabe, M.D. is a board certified psychiatrist currently living in Wausau, WI. She obtained her medical degree from the Chicago Medical School in 1983 and went on to complete her psychiatric residency in 1988 at the University of Michigan in Ann Arbor, MI. Dr. Wohlrabe practiced medicine for many years as an adult and adolescent psychiatrist before taking on the role as Medical Director for Aspirus Wausau Hospital's Eating Disorders Program in Wausau, Wisconsin. When she retired from the program in order to more fully devote herself to her family, her psychiatric interests evolved to focus on individuals who would not typically step foot in an eating disorders clinic - the average person who secretly and quietly struggles with disordered eating and weight management. Dr. Wohlrabe decided to write *Healthy & Lean: The Science of Metabolism and the Psychology of Weight Management* because she passionately believes that the moms, dads, athletes, college students, ballerinas, CEOs, teachers, nurses and children of this world - in short, *everyone* - deserves to be equipped with the nutritional knowledge and psychological tools that will lead to satisfaction and success.

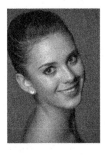

Ileana Riverón is an experienced writer and researcher who became passionate about nutritional education during her years as a professional ballerina. While dancing in Florida, London and Boston, she witnessed the far-reaching effects of the ballet community's ongoing struggle with body dissatisfaction and eating disorders and determined to effect positive change. She went on to study at Harvard University and was honored as one of fifteen members of the prestigious Mount Vernon Leadership Fellowship in 2015. There, she worked with specialists from the Empowered Eating Blog and the Eating Disorders Coalition for Research, Policy and Action to innovate eating disorders prevention and recovery initiatives. Ileana has given talks and deepened the academic literature on this topic with guidance from faculty members of the Harvard T.H. Chan School of Public Health and Harvard Medical School. Combining her love of writing and her insight into the spectrum of disordered eating, Ileana has enjoyed acting as research assistant and co-author of *Healthy & Lean: The Science of Metabolism and the Psychology of Weight Management*. She hopes this book will prove to be a fun and accessible guide to healthy living for any reader.

CPSIA information can be obtained
at www.ICGtesting.com
Printed in the USA
BVOW05s1453100117
473118BV00001BB/9/P